Analysis of hospital costs:
a manual for managers

Donald S. Shepard
Dominic Hodgkin
Yvonne E. Anthony

Institute for Health Policy
Heller Graduate School
Brandeis University
Waltham, MA, USA

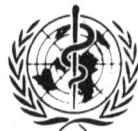

World Health Organization
Geneva
2000

WHO Library Cataloguing-in-Publication Data

Shepard, Donald S.
    Analysis of hospital costs : a manual for managers / Donald S. Shepard,
    Dominic Hodgkin, Yvonne E. Anthony.

    1.Economics, Hospital   2.Financial management, Hospital   3.Costs and cost analysis
    4.Administrative personnel   5.Manuals   I.Hodgkin, Dominic   II.Anthony, Yvonne E.
    III.Title

    ISBN 92 4 154528 3   (NLM Classifications: WX 157)

The World Health Organization welcomes requests for permission to reproduce or translate its publications, in part or in full. Applications and enquiries should be addressed to the Office of Publications, World Health Organization, Geneva, Switzerland, which will be glad to provide the latest information on any changes made to the text, plans for new editions, and reprints and translations already available.

The designations employed and the presentation of the material in this publication do not imply the expression of any opinion whatsoever on the part of the Secretariat of the World Health Organization concerning the legal status of any country, territory, city or area or of its authorities, or concerning the delimitation of its frontiers or boundaries.

The mention of specific companies or of certain manufacturers' products does not imply that they are endorsed or recommended by the World Health Organization in preference to others of a similar nature that are not mentioned. Errors and omissions excepted, the names of proprietary products are distinguished by initial capital letters.

The authors alone are responsible for the views expressed in this publication.

Typeset in Hong Kong
Printed in Singapore

98/12345 — Best-set/SNP — 6000

Contents

Preface

Consideration of cost takes an increasing amount of the attention of managers in health facilities and at district, regional and national levels of the health service. This concern applies in both the public and private (including both for-profit and not-for-profit) sectors. In 1994, in collaboration with UNICEF and the Aga Khan Foundation, WHO published *Cost analysis in primary health care*[1] to strengthen the management of primary health care programmes. Hospitals absorb the bulk of health spending in most countries, however, and the evidence suggests that there is considerable scope for improving the management of these resources. That is why this manual was prepared. A draft was completed in early 1997 and its usefulness to managers was tested through workshops in Bangladesh and Zimbabwe that year, and in Egypt in 1999. The present publication incorporates feedback from the workshop participants.

This manual is intended to help managers at various levels of the health system understand how cost analysis can assist decision-making, as well as to help them define and institutionalize relevant costing systems. The manual gives methodological guidance and it is expected that each country can and should develop its own costing strategy and specific methodologies on the basis of managerial needs and the availability of relevant information. It is hoped that the manual will facilitate national processes for developing hospital costing strategies and methods.

---

[1] Creese A, Parker D, eds. *Cost analysis in primary health care: a training manual for programme managers.* Geneva, World Health Organization, 1994.

Acknowledgements

The field tests of the draft versions of this book in Bangladesh and Zimbabwe were coordinated by James Killingsworth and Thomas Zigora, respectively, and were supported by the British Department for International Development (DFID). Both the Danish International Development Agency (DANIDA) and the US Agency for International Development (USAID) have contributed to WHO's activities in the area of hospital cost analysis including the Interregional Workshop on Hospital Cost Analysis held in Egypt in 1999.

The authors wish to thank the many people who provided them with advice, knowledge and relevant background documents, particularly Joseph Kutzin of the WHO Department of Evidence for Health Policy who gave them information on numerous studies and invaluable feedback on an earlier draft. They also express their thanks to Guy Carrin of the WHO Department of Health in Sustainable Development, Andrew Creese of the WHO Department of Evidence for Health Policy, and Claudio Politi, consultant, for their helpful comments, and to the authors of several studies referenced in this book who made their work available.

About the authors

Donald S. Shepard Ph.D. is Research Professor at the Institute of Health Policy, Heller Graduate School, Brandeis University, Waltham MA, USA. His research focuses on cost-effectiveness analysis, health insurance and managed care, both internationally and in the United States of America.

Dominic Hodgkin Ph.D. is Senior Research Associate at the Institute of Health Policy, Heller Graduate School, Brandeis University, Waltham, MA, USA. He conducts research on economic issues in health care, particularly mental health and substance abuse.

Yvonne E. Anthony Ph.D. is Senior Research Associate and Adjunct Lecturer at the Institute of Health Policy, Heller Graduate School, Brandeis University, Waltham, MA, USA. Her research focuses on cost of and access to services under managed care.

Introduction

Purpose of this manual

According to a major World Bank study of public hospitals (Barnum & Kutzin, 1993), the share of public sector health resources consumed by hospitals in developing countries ranges from 50% to 80%. This manual seeks to help health facility and health system managers to make the best use of these resources. Thus, the target audience includes hospital managers (both financial and programmatic), public sector managers at the district, regional and national levels of the health system, and persons responsible for non-profit and private hospital systems. By better understanding the costs of various activities, managers can improve the efficiency of hospital departments, as well as hospital systems as a whole. The data can also help national policy-makers to decide which curative care is best delivered in hospitals and to examine the trade-offs between various preventive, primary curative and secondary curative services.

The type of information available for cost analysis in countries and hospitals varies from extensive to rudimentary. Hospitals vary in the extent to which costs are allocated to specific hospital departments and in the accuracy with which such allocations are recorded. In light of this, the manual spells out alternative approaches wherever possible and suggests which approaches can be taken when information is incomplete.

The manual provides a framework for both deriving and analysing hospital costs. Chapter 1 shows how to compute unit costs. Since data may often be incomplete, the chapter also shows how cost allocations between cost centres can be imputed from staffing data or approximated from other available information. Complementary information from each department can be obtained by interviewing hospital personnel (e.g. staff time, wages, allowances, supplies, space occupied, activities performed) or by extracting data from management information systems or medical records (e.g. amounts of care provided). Chapters 2 and 3 apply knowledge gained from the previous chapter by discussing ways in which cost data can be utilized at the level of the individual hospital (Chapter 2) or the hospital system (Chapter 3). In many small hospitals in developing countries, costs may not be reported at all by individual departments or reporting may be very incomplete or arbitrary. Thus, Chapter 3 shows how to compute unit costs when line item data are completely missing or not usable. Since managers of various units of the health system are concerned with different parts of the system, it is expected that many readers will consult this manual selectively and concentrate only on the components that apply to them. The manual has been used in workshops in Bangladesh, Egypt and Zimbabwe. Appendix 4 contains case studies based on those workshops. The workshops proved to be a stimulating format for introducing the topics in this manual and encouraging managers to think more broadly about strengthening their institutions. The case studies can be used to facilitate that process.

Cost-finding and cost analysis as management tools

In both developing and developed countries, hospitals are seen as vital and necessary community resources that should be managed for the benefit of the community (World Health Organization, 1987, 1992; Van Lerberghe & Lafort, 1990; Institute for Health Policy Studies, 1996). As such, hospital management has a responsibility to the community to provide health care services that the community needs at an acceptable level of quality and at the least possible cost. Cost-finding and analysis can help departmental managers, hospital administrators and policy-makers to determine how well their institutions meet these public needs.

Cost-finding and cost analysis are techniques for allocating direct and indirect costs, as explained in this manual. They are also the means of manipulating or rearranging the data or information in existing accounts in order to obtain the costs of services rendered by the hospital. As financial management techniques, cost-finding and cost analysis help to furnish the necessary data for making more informed decisions on operations and infrastructure investments. If structured accurately, cost data can provide information on operational performance by cost centre. This information can be compared to budgeted performance expectations in order to identify problem areas that require immediate attention. These data give management the material to evaluate and modify operations if necessary. Moreover, knowledge of costs (both unit and total) can assist in planning of future budgets (as an indicator of efficiency) and in establishing a schedule of charges for patient services. A hospital cannot set rates and charges that are realistically related to costs unless the cost-finding system accurately allocates both direct and indirect costs to the appropriate cost centre.

Finally, cost-finding and cost analysis are also of value to management in ensuring that costs do not exceed available revenues and subsidies. They are the best techniques available for accomplishing this.

Chapter 1

Computing unit costs using line item expenditure data

Two fundamental items of financial data needed by a hospital manager are allocated costs by cost centre (a programme or department within a hospital) and the unit cost of hospital services. A unit of hospital services may be as small as one meal or as broad as an entire inpatient stay. This chapter explains how to allocate costs by cost centre and how to compute unit costs. To perform these calculations precisely, the hospital needs an accurate and comprehensive financial accounting system. In many hospitals, however, existing accounting systems have gaps, in that some costs are excluded or the data are lacking to enable costs to be related to specific cost centres. In such cases, estimates are needed. This chapter provides a number of suggestions for generating such approximations. It follows seven steps for computing unit costs, built on the procedures of the UNICEF manual for analysis of district health service costs and financing (Hanson & Gilson, 1996).[1] The steps are as follows:

1. Define the final product.
2. Define cost centres.
3. Identify the full cost for each input.
4. Assign inputs to cost centres.
5. Allocate all costs to final cost centres (compute total allocated costs).
6. Compute unit cost for each final cost centre.
7. Report results.

In leading the reader through these steps, the present manual explains what data elements are needed, how different cost items can be treated, and how costs can be computed in certain situations or cases. In each case, there is discussion of a set of problems that have been identified in various studies of specific countries (see Table 1).[2] In addition, examples of certain points are discussed in more detail (see Boxes 2 to 5 and Tables A1 to A5).

---

[1] The presentation of the steps in this manual differs slightly from the nine steps presented by Hanson & Gilson for costing district hospitals, but the concepts and methodologies are consistent with each other.

[2] The principal studies are listed in Table 1 in alphabetical order by country. Full citations are provided in the references on pages 60–63. For a review of the findings of some of these studies, see Barnum & Kutzin (1993).

Table 1. Selected studies of hospital costs

Country	Authors	Title	Year
Algeria	Djelloul B	Hôpital specialisé en maladies infectieuses d'El-Kettar (Alger)	no date
Belize	Raymond S et al.	Financing and costs of health services in Belize	1987
Bhutan (I)	Huff-Rousselle M	Financial study of Thimphu General Hospital	1992
Bhutan (II)	Huff-Rousselle M	Dzongkhag costing study for Tashigang Dzongkhag	1992
Bolivia	Olave M, Montano Z	Unit cost and financial analysis for the Hospital *12 de abril* in Bolivia	1993
Colombia	Robertson R et al.	Hospital cost accounting and analysis: the case of Candelaria	1977
Dominica	Gill L	Hospital costing study: Princess Margaret Hospital	1994
Dominican Republic	Lewis M et al.	Measuring public hospital costs: empirical evidence from the Dominican Republic	1995
Ecuador	LaForgia G, Balarezo M	Cost recovery in public sector hospitals in Ecuador	1993
Egypt (I)	Zaman S	Cost analysis for hospital care	1993
Egypt (II)	Salah H	Cost analysis for hospital care: summary output	1996
Gambia	Ministry of Health/WHO	Cost analysis of the health care sector in the Gambia	1995
Guinea	Carrin G, Evlo K	A methodology for the calculation of health care costs and their recovery	1995
Indonesia	RAND Corporation	Unit cost analysis: a manual for facility administrators and policy-makers	1992
Jamaica	Kutzin J	Jamaican hospital restoration project: final report	1989
Lesotho	Puglisi R, Bicknell WJ	Functional expenditure analysis: final report for Queen Elizabeth II Hospital	1990
Malawi	Mills A	The cost of the district hospital: a case study from Malawi	1991
Montserrat	Gill L, Percy A	Hospital costing study: Glendon Hospital, Montserrat	1994
Namibia	Bamako Initiative Management Unit	Cost, resource use and financing of district health services	1994
Niger	Wong H	Cost analysis of Niamey Hospital	1989
Papua New Guinea	John Snow, Inc.	Papua New Guinea: health sector financing study project	1990
Russian Federation	Telyukov A	A guide to methodology: integrated system of cost accounting and analysis for inpatient care providers	1995
Rwanda	Shepard DS	Analysis and recommendations on health financing in Rwanda	1988
St Lucia	Russell S et al.	Victoria Hospital	1988
Sierra Leone	Ojo K et al.	Cost analysis of health services in Sierra Leone	1995
Tuvalu	Wong H	Health financing in Tuvalu	1993
Zimbabwe	Bijlmakers L, Chihanga S	District health service costs, resource adequacy and efficiency: a comparison of three districts	1996

Defining the final product of the cost analysis

What are the services or departments for which you are interested in computing unit costs? For example, do you want to know the unit cost for all inpatient services, or do you want a separate unit cost figure for each ward or service? The decision will depend on two key factors:

- *Purpose of the analysis.* If you want to do a comparison of costs of certain hospital departments, you will want to compute unit costs for each department separately.[1] If you want to compare multiple hospitals with similar caseloads (e.g. all district hospitals within a particular state or region), it may be sufficient to compute a single unit cost for all inpatient care for each hospital.
- *Type of data available.* Your ability to compute unit costs will be constrained by how aggregate or disaggregate the available data are for both costs and utilization. For example, in order to compute unit costs by ward, one would at least need to have utilization data by ward (e.g. actual total patient-days for each ward for a particular budget year). If these data cannot be identified by ward, it will make more sense to compute unit costs at the next higher level (e.g. all inpatient wards or units that house internal medicine patients or surgery patients).

In some cases, it may be unclear whether to compute a separate unit cost for a certain activity or allocate its costs to some other output. For example, some studies have computed separate unit costs for laboratory and radiology departments, thereby excluding those costs from the cost per inpatient-day or per discharge. Others have treated laboratory and radiology as intermediate outputs and fully allocated their costs to the inpatient cost centres. Again, the desirability of each approach depends on the purpose of the analysis, but it is important to be consistent. It may even be desirable to report results in both forms (as was done in the Lesotho study listed in Table 1).

For each final cost centre (see pages 4–5 for descriptions of types of cost centres), one must define the unit of output (e.g. inpatient-day, admission, visit). For inpatient care, the usual choices are inpatient-days or admissions. For outpatient care, number of visits is the unit of output. A variety of other output units have been used for other cost centres. Examples include the number of tests or examinations (for laboratory and X-ray departments), the number of operations (for operating theatres) and the number of prescriptions (for pharmacy departments).

One can analyse unit cost based on data for a single month, a quarter-year or a year. The data period chosen will depend first on how the available data are organized. Sometimes important data such as utility costs (e.g. fuel, water, electricity) are available only on an annual basis; to do a quarterly analysis, one would have to make assumptions about use patterns during the year.

---

[1] See Chapters 2 and 3 for a fuller discussion of the purposes of unit costing.

In such situations, it may make more sense to analyse data for a whole year rather than for each quarter.

A second consideration in the choice of data period is the purpose of the analysis. If managers are trying to understand a rapid recent change in costs, then quarterly or monthly analysis may be appropriate. However, if the aim is to compare one hospital's costs to those of other hospitals, or to compare fees paid by patients treated in similar health care settings, it may make more sense to use a longer period of time. Using annual data may help to "equalize seasonal variations" since each hospital is affected by these factors differently.

Defining cost centres

The next step for computing unit costs is to determine the centres of activity in the hospital to which direct and/or indirect costs will be assigned. The major direct cost categories of most departments include salaries, supplies and other (purchased services, travel and rents). Indirect cost categories include depreciation and allocated costs of other departments.

The rationale for choosing centres of activity that correspond with the hospital's organizational and/or accounting structure is managerial. Hospitals are organized into departments and, since the aim is to strengthen the management of these departments, it is useful to have cost centres that correspond to the organizational structure of the hospital. This provides a route map by which costs can be channelled through the process of cost-finding to final cost centres, and a framework for costing the distinct functions of each centre. Following this route map shows individual managers how they are using available resources in relation to what has been budgeted and the services that they are providing.

Some cost centres represent patient-centred activities (i.e. final or intermediate cost centres), while others are primarily for general services (i.e. overhead cost centres) such as housekeeping, laundry, maintenance and the many other tasks necessary for the satisfactory operation of a complex organization like a hospital. From an administrative standpoint, cost centres can be distinguished according to the nature of their work — patient care, intermediate clinical care, and overhead centres.

- *Patient care.* These cost centres are responsible for direct patient services such as wards or inpatient care units as a whole, or the ambulatory care centre.
- *Intermediate.* These cost centres provide ancillary services to support patient care units but are organized as separate departments. Examples include laboratory, pharmacy and radiology.
- *Overhead.* These cost centres provide overhead support services to both patient care and intermediate cost centres. Examples of overhead departments are finance (accounts receivable, accounts payable, payroll, etc.), dietetics and security.

Within each of the above groups, decisions also have to be made about how many cost centres to define. For instance, if you are planning to analyse unit costs by ward, you would need to treat each ward as a separate cost centre. Or, if you want to distinguish ancillary costs by type (e.g. X-ray department versus clinical laboratory), you would need to establish separate cost centres for each.

The aim of unit cost analysis is to allocate hospital costs (direct and indirect) to centres whose costs are to be measured. Typically, you will be computing the unit cost mainly for patient care centres (e.g. maternity wards, outpatient clinics, paediatric units). However, in some instances you may need to know the cost per laboratory test or per drug prescription, in which case unit costs are computed for intermediate departments such as laboratory and pharmacy. On occasion, you may even need to know the unit cost of an overhead service such as dietetics if, for example, you are considering opening a competitive bidding process to contract food services rather than keeping it in-house, or if you wish to compare the performance of dietetic departments in different hospitals.

In order to see the extent to which user charges (e.g. fees for room, board, and nursing [a daily rate inclusive of diagnostic and therapeutic services], drugs and dressings, X-ray, laboratory, physical therapy) cover their associated costs, it may be necessary to have a cost analysis system that identifies cost centres which produce revenue (i.e. patient care and intermediate cost centres) and general cost centres that do not produce revenue (e.g. security, housekeeping, payroll). This identification is necessary when it is desirable to allocate all direct or indirect expenses incurred by the general cost centre (non-revenue-producing centres) to revenue-producing centres which could be the final cost centres.

Finally, one may eventually want to compute two types of unit costs: with or without allocated ancillary amounts. For example, when calculating the cost per admission or inpatient stay, one figure could include laboratory and X-ray costs and one could exclude them (see the Lesotho study by Puglisi & Bicknell, 1990, for a discussion of both types of unit cost).

Identifying the full cost for each input

An important part of computing unit costs is to make sure that you have cost data which are as complete as possible. Two issues are involved: the conceptual issue of determining which expenditures should be counted as costs based on an economic sense of resources used up during the production of health care, and the actual measurement of true costs using available data (which may be incomplete or untrustworthy). Various studies have developed ways to impute or approximate cost when existing data are problematic, and some of these are described. Since the problems and responses often differ according to the line item, the discussion is partly organized by line item (e.g. salaries, drugs).

Salaries

To calculate the full or total cost of salaries, one should ideally use actual salary amounts paid to hospital employees. Sometimes these data may not be available at the hospital, as in situations where employees are paid by the Ministry of Health or Ministry of Public Service, and therefore the hospital cannot access payroll data directly. However, as some studies have shown, individual salaries can be approximated by using the midpoint of the salary range of the employee's classification level. In Mills' study on hospitals in Malawi, the midpoint estimation approach appeared reasonable given that the estimated total wage costs were similar to the hospital's true wage costs. On the other hand, another study has shown that using the midpoint estimation approach may not accurately reflect true salaries. Researchers in Niger obtained data on the mean salary for each job classification across all hospitals and found it was consistently lower than the midpoint, often by as much as 30%. Reanalysing their data, we determined that using the midpoint in this study would have overstated true payroll cost by around 35%.

In some hospitals, salary information on certain expatriate staff may be hard to obtain if they are paid by foreign donor agencies with salaries denominated in foreign currency. However, some studies have costed these staff using local physicians' wages, arguing that, if the expatriate staff leave, they would be replaced by local physicians. The validity of this approach depends on the purpose of the costing analysis. If the aim is to project future budget/resource needs after the expatriates leave, then using local wage rates is appropriate. However, if the goal is to estimate current unit costs, local wages may understate the true cost of resources used, depending on the currency exchange rate and differences between expatriate and local wages. Thus, the rationale behind the costing analysis will suggest which measure is most appropriate.

In some cases, individuals may be employed and paid by more than one hospital. If so, the proportion of their time spent in each hospital must be determined and applied accordingly. For example, if an employee spends four days working in your hospital and one day a week elsewhere, then you should be paying only 80% of his/her salary and the other facility should pay the remaining 20%. The same rationale should be applied to fringe benefits.

Fringe benefits

In principle, fringe benefits (e.g. health care insurance, vacation, sick pay, dental care) received by personnel as part of their employment should be included as part of total payroll costs. This is true whether these benefits are paid by the hospital, by public sector funds managed by the Ministry of Health, or by both. Examples of such benefits are "gratuities" to physicians (the St Lucia study) and employees' share of hospital fees or revenues (the Niger study).

To obtain a full and accurate picture of personnel costs of a hospital, one may need to know not only the cost of paid salaries and fringe benefits but, for planning purposes, also the "in-kind costs" (such as unpaid work or voluntary work). In a hospital study in Colombia, Robertson and colleagues measured unpaid work along with fringe benefits and determined that both accounted for 40% of true personnel costs (or 30% of total direct costs). They measured unpaid work by using outside observers to monitor staff activities and record time-study measurements for each employee. An example of unpaid work is time spent treating patients beyond normal clinic hours because of physician or nursing inefficiencies, overbookings and/or missed appointments. By not including unpaid labour when determining levels of productivity or efficiency, programme managers or planners may reach an erroneous conclusion.

Donated items

Typically, when materials and equipment have been provided by foreign donors, they will not appear in hospital spending records. However, since the hospital is using these donated items, they should be included in calculations of hospital unit costs. This is especially relevant for regional or national health authorities responsible for comparing the performance of different hospitals. If the value of donated inputs is not included in the cost analysis, hospitals or wards with more donated items may appear more efficient than others, even though their actual efficiency may be the same. Such items can account for a substantial share of hospital resources. In a study in Niger, for example, donated drugs amounted to 19% of total drug spending and donated food to 20% of total food spending.

The treatment of donated capital items is discussed later. This section considers donated recurrent items — i.e. those used up within the period of analysis. Examples would be bandages and syringes. The correct costing procedure is to prepare a list of these items and find out the replacement cost of each (i.e. what it would now cost to purchase them).

It is worth explaining the reasons for costing donated items since they may not apply in all situations. First, donated items may have an "opportunity cost" — i.e. one may want to consider how productive they would be if transferred to a different ward or hospital from the one where they currently happen to be used. This issue is less relevant if the donation cannot be transferred (e.g. due to restrictions imposed by the donor) and the ministry cannot reallocate funds toward hospitals which receive fewer donations (e.g. due to "maintenance of effort" restrictions imposed by donors). The second reason to cost donated items is that, at some point, donations may dry up or a long-lived donated item may need replacing. The hospital needs to anticipate these possibilities. The third reason is to avoid penalizing hospitals that look inefficient compared to others merely because they receive fewer donations.

Ministry of Health spending

In many countries, the Ministry of Health pays directly for some resources used by hospitals (e.g. stationery, vehicle maintenance, salaries). This arrangement poses no special problem if the ministry keeps records on how funding was allocated to hospitals. When this is the case, one needs only to add allocations to the appropriate expenditure line items.

However, sometimes the ministry cannot determine specific spending levels by hospital. In this case, one will need to estimate the allocated amounts by line item oneself, preferably in consultation with officials at the hospital and the ministry. For example, in Tuvalu, most spending on the single hospital came from the ministry's budget and was not distinguished from spending on health centres. The study authors estimated the hospital's share for each line item after discussion with those involved. These discussions suggested that, for example, the hospital accounted for 100% of laboratory costs, 90% of electricity and 80% of medical supplies. These suggested percentages were applied to the national expenditure data and the resulting figures were assigned to the hospital.

Drugs

Sometimes spending data on drugs and other consumable medical supplies are not available from the hospital's own accounts or from those of the central ministry. For example, in some countries, drugs are purchased by a centralized government agency which then supplies them to hospitals without this appearing in the Ministry of Health or hospital budget. In such cases, it is necessary to access the agency's records and determine the value of drugs shipped to the hospital(s) of interest. Sometimes (as in the Papua New Guinea study) the central agency can provide a printout of the value of shipments. In other cases, only quantities are reported, in which case the value of the drugs can be computed by obtaining the price paid for each drug item and multiplying this figure by the respective quantity.

If the agency recorded which departments within each hospital ordered or received the drugs, this information will be important at later stages of the cost analysis and should be included in any transfer of data.

The large volume of drug data may make it impractical to analyse a full year's data. In some studies, consultants analysed a sample of pharmacy records rather than data for a full year. In fact, to estimate one year's use, the St Lucia study used a two-month sample of pharmacy requisitions from the central medical stores. If this approach is taken, one should try to sample various points in the year to account for seasonal variations in drug utilization.

As in the case of Mills' Malawi study, the hospital pharmacy can have information on drug deliveries to each ward but may not know the value or price of the drugs. If this is because drugs are paid for by a centralized government agency, one can ask the agency the price it pays for each of the drugs concerned and evaluate drug consumption using those prices.

Fuel

If records of spending on fuel are not available, it may be possible to estimate spending indirectly. Some hospitals keep logbooks for personnel to record distance travelled by each vehicle on each trip. By estimating the distance travelled per unit of fuel (e.g. miles per gallon) or the amount of fuel needed to cover a certain distance (e.g. litres per 100 km), one can further calculate the total fuel consumed over a given period. In turn, spending on fuel can be estimated by valuing the fuel consumption at the local retail price per gallon or litre.

Similarly, spending figures may not be available for generators and other hospital equipment. As in the case of the WHO Gambia study, spending can be estimated using information about how often the equipment is used, the rate at which it consumes fuel and the price per unit of fuel.

Maintenance

In some countries, personnel who maintain public hospitals are employed by the Ministry of Health rather than by the individual hospital. This might lead one to understate the true cost of operating the hospital. As with other centrally supplied inputs (such as drugs), the question is whether the central agency can report how much service it provided to each hospital. If not, one must devise a rule to allocate some portion of the central maintenance budget to each hospital being studied. The simplest way would be to assume that the hospital's share of maintenance costs is proportional to its area (square feet or metres). A more accurate approach might then be to weigh older hospitals more heavily, on the assumption that they need more intensive maintenance.

Spending from user fee revenue

A common component of many cost recovery programmes is to allow the hospital to retain a portion of fees charged. For example, in the Jamaican hospitals studied by Kutzin, hospitals were allowed to keep 50% of revenues generated. Spending of retained revenues may be hard to measure, especially if financial controls are poor. Yet it is important to try, given the growing significance of this source of revenue in many poor countries.

In some countries the amount of revenues retained (or of costs recovered) is not well documented. If this is the case, one can estimate retained revenues by applying the fee schedule to available utilization data. For example, if the hospital charges 10 francs per outpatient visit and 50 francs per inpatient-day, and if there are 1000 outpatient visits and 1000 inpatient-days monthly, then the total fee revenue for that time period would be 60000 francs

([10 × 1000] + [50 × 1000]). If some patients received free care due to their inability to pay or because their fees were not collected, total cost recovery would be overstated if this fact were not taken into account.

Having estimated total cost recovery, one can determine how the money was spent by line item or cost centre. Even if hospital records do not indicate uses of fee revenues, interviews with staff may shed light on this question. For example, through staff interviews, Kutzin concluded that the Jamaican hospitals were spending much of their revenue fees on "breakdown" maintenance.

A further complication exists in hospitals where staff are practising unofficial cost recovery without transmitting the proceeds to the hospital accounts. Ojo and colleagues estimated these amounts to be substantial in the Sierra Leone hospitals which they studied. Even if one can measure these amounts, their treatment depends on how one thinks they are being spent and the purpose of the analysis. If staff are spending the money to buy supplies, then these are costs of the hospital and should be included in a cost analysis (if measurable). If the unofficial fees are being treated as private income by staff, and are spent outside the hospital, then they should not be included in a hospital cost analysis. On the other hand, the amounts collected may be relevant to a cost recovery analysis, as they indicate patients' willingness to pay, which might be better exploited by the hospital itself than by its staff.

Delayed payments

As in conventional accounting analysis, cost measures may be misstated when services are paid in a different accounting period from that in which they are used. The Jamaica study by Kutzin found large fluctuations in utility payments which did not reflect real resource use even within a fiscal year. This occurred because some hospitals were able to delay payment for months and then make large settlements later. The study author corrected for this by using actual kilowatt-hours when available, and otherwise using hospitals' budget requests for utilities. Without the correction, the same facility would have shown variations over time in calculated unit cost, which would be difficult to explain.

Capital items

Capital assets are assets that have an economically useful life exceeding one year and that are not acquired primarily for resale. A unit cost analysis which ignores capital is essentially assuming that the present physical assets will be available for ever. In reality, assets are being worn down by the hospital's daily activities, and this depreciation is an expense. Unlike drug purchases or salaries, however, depreciation is not an expenditure; it does not require an actual cost outlay. Therefore, depreciation may be hard to measure if certain information is not available (such as purchase price and the useful life of its equipment). If this is the case, then determining the depreciation expense becomes more sensitive to the analyst's assumptions.

For the present analysis, we are not necessarily trying to compute a "depreciation allowance" or find how much to save up for equipment replacement. Rather, the aim is to estimate the opportunity cost of the capital being used up, and to do so in a way that is consistent across periods. Reflecting this, the methodology we present here differs somewhat from more familiar accounting-based approaches.

To measure the cost of eventually replacing capital, several questions must be answered for each asset (see Box 1 for an example of the calculation of annual capital costs).

What is the asset's total life? A typical assumption for a building is a total life of 30 years. Other studies have assumed that beds and furniture last 10 years and that vehicles last five years. The assumption matters most for items with a large share of cost, such as buildings, vehicles and major medical equipment.

What will be the cost of replacing the asset at the end of the year? Financial accounts often calculate depreciation on the basis of an asset's original purchase price (historic cost). However, if there is inflation (as in most countries), historic cost will understate the amount required to replace a given asset. Replacement cost is the more relevant measure for those planning resource use.

From this viewpoint, the original purchase cost is useful only as a starting point for working out the cost of replacing the asset. Of course, even the original cost may not be available (if it was donated). If an estimate of original cost is made, it must be updated to the present year and each future year in which replacement could occur. In other words, one must forecast the inflation that is likely to occur from now until the year of replacement. Estimates of local inflation are often available from governments or aid agencies for a number of years ahead but become increasingly unavailable (and unreliable) beyond five years.

If the replacement must be paid for with foreign currency, one should also predict how the cost of foreign currency (i.e. the exchange rate) will change over the period in question. Sometimes exchange rate forecasts are available from the central bank, or one can extrapolate from recent experience. In the Gambia study, the authors assumed an annual exchange rate deterioration of 27%.

What interest rate should be applied to money saved now for future replacement? Calculations of a "capital cost" typically apply some kind of interest rate based on that which would be paid on a local savings account. This is often justified by imagining that the hospital is saving up to replace its equipment and can deposit the savings in an interest-bearing account. This approach has been criticized as unrealistic in many developing countries where public hospitals lack the authority to deposit funds in this way.

Box 1. Example of how to compute annual capital cost

Table 2 provides data for this example of how to compute annual capital cost on two assets, one available locally and one which must be imported. Each was purchased 10 years ago and has 10 years of useful life remaining. The answers to the standard questions are as follows:

1. Total life of the asset: 20 years.

2. Replacement cost: to replace each asset at today's prices would cost 1000 francs (the local currency). The price of locally produced items is increasing at 3% per year. However, the gradual devaluation of the local currency means that prices of imported goods rise at a faster rate, namely 4% per year.

3. Real interest rate: this depends on the nominal interest rate and the inflation rate. Therefore, in this example, the real interest rate differs for the two assets.

Using these assumptions, the hospital can compute a reasonable measure of its annual capital cost using the following formula:

Capital cost in year k = (Replacement cost in year k ÷ annualization factor)

The annualization factor is defined on the basis of the real interest rate and the total life of the asset. Values are provided in Appendix 3.

For the first asset, the real interest rate is computed as

real r = (1 + nominal interest rate) ÷ (1 + annual inflation) − 1
       = (1.06 − 1.03) − 1
       = 0.0291

So the real interest rate is 2.9%. This can be rounded to 3% for this example. Indeed, a real interest rate of 3% has been applied to a range of countries.

Appendix 3 gives the annualization factor for a 3% real interest rate and a life of 20 years. The annualization factor is 14.877.

The replacement cost next year will be 1030 francs, since 3% inflation will have occurred. Dividing by the annualization factor, the capital cost for next year is therefore 69.23 francs. The following year's capital cost is similarly computed as 71 francs (1060.90 ÷ 14.877). The capital cost therefore increases from year to year at the rate of inflation. (Capital cost computed in this way stays constant in real terms.)

If one needs to consider a discount rate or time period that is not provided in Appendix 3, one can compute the annualization factor using the formula:

Factor = (l ÷ r) × [1 − (1 ÷ (1+r)^n)]

where r is the real interest rate and n is the number of years of life.

Thus, the capital cost this year is 69 francs, and this becomes part of the hospital's costs to be allocated across cost centres in a full step-down analysis.

For the second asset, the annual inflation is higher (4%). In the first year, replacement would cost 1040 francs (1000 × 1.04), so the capital cost in that year is 69.90 francs (1040 ÷ 14.877), and it increases in subsequent years at the rate of inflation in the foreign asset's price.

Note: If instead one took the first asset's original purchase cost of 744 francs and depreciated it over 20 years on a straight-line basis, the annual depreciation for each asset would be 37 francs (i.e. 744 divided by 20). This approach would understate the true opportunity cost of the capital being used up, since it ignores inflation in the purchase price.

Table 2. Data for worked example of annual capital cost[a,b]

	Beginning of this year	End of this year	End of next year
Total useful life (years)	20	20	20
Annualization factor	14.877	14.877	14.877
Domestic asset			
Replacement cost	1000.00	1030.00	1060.90
Annual capital cost	n.a.	69.23	71.31
Foreign asset			
Replacement cost	1000.00	1040.00	1081.60
Annual capital cost	n.a.	69.91	72.70

[a] For interpretation, see Box 1.
[b] Assumes interest paid annually at end of year.
n.a. = not applicable.

The method proposed here continues to use the real (inflation-free) interest rate, but it is justified by imagining that the hospital could rent medical equipment instead of buying it. To find the maximum rental payment the hospital should be willing to make, one would use this same approach (assuming perfect capital markets).

Box 1 provides an example of these calculations for two assets — one which can be purchased with local currency and one which must be imported.

Finally, given the uncertainty associated with measurements of capital costs, it may be advisable to present two sets of results, one including capital cost and one excluding it. This approach was taken by Ojo and colleagues in Sierra Leone. Their results showed that including capital costs substantially increased unit costs on inpatient wards (by 30–50%) but had little effect on unit costs of the operating room. This appears to be because the wards had more valuable equipment and, in most cases, more floor space than the operating theatre.

In general, we suggest using a real interest rate of 3%. This rate has been found in many industrialized and developing economies. As this rate was used in a comprehensive set of cost–effectiveness studies for the health sector (Jamison et al., 1993), its use makes hospital costing consistent with the international literature.

Assigning inputs to cost centres

At this point, information has been gathered about the hospital's total costs, whatever the source of payment. This information alone may provide useful insights even before one starts computing unit costs: for instance, in identifying which line items account for most of the cost and whether this is changing over time (see Box 2). However, to compute unit costs one must proceed to the next step: assigning costs from each line item to the relevant cost centres.

Box 2. Worked example for a hypothetical hospital

This box is the first in a series which works through an example of unit costing for a hypothetical hospital. Table A1 (page 64) lists the hospital's costs by line item, such as salary and drugs, and by source of payment. Although most costs (70%) are paid by the Ministry of Health, other payment sources are also important. Donors pay for one physician's salary and for half of "other supplies", while a government drug agency pays for drug shipments. Failure to include these other payment sources (e.g. by omitting drugs) would both understate total cost and misrepresent the true distribution of spending.

Even if one does not compute unit costs, drawing up a table like this can by itself provide helpful information. It shows the relative importance of the different payment sources and where the contributions of each are concentrated. Comparisons with previous years may help identify problems or trends (e.g. declining donor support or spiralling drug purchase costs).

Some inputs can be assigned directly to certain cost centres. For instance, if "kitchen" is a cost centre, then the line item "food" could be assigned to that cost centre. More often, inputs are used by several cost centres and the analyst must seek to assign spending for an input across those centres. Correct assignment is most important for those inputs which account for a larger share of costs, such as staff time and drugs. For an illustration, see Box 3.

Staff time

Various methods have been used to assign staff time to cost centres, ranging from simple (using administrative data) to elaborate (direct measurement).

Administrative data

Many hospitals have duty rosters showing which staff are assigned to which departments. Since many staff typically work in only one department, the roster can be used to allocate these staff. Those who work in several departments can be interviewed individually, although this may be time-consuming if there are many of them. Alternatively, the manager can be asked how many hours each works in each department, and salaries (and fringe benefits) can be allocated pro rata accordingly.

Direct measurement

The Dominican Republic study by Lewis and colleagues used the most comprehensive approach to allocating staff time. They employed data collectors who followed medical staff over a period of weeks and recorded the time

---

> ### Box 3. Cost assignment in the worked example
>
> Table A2 (page 65) takes the cost data for the hypothetical Hospital X (from Table A1), and shows how the line items can be assigned to cost centres. The aim here is to obtain unit costs for the three wards: medical, surgical and maternity. Data on salaries, drugs and supplies must be assigned to the wards and to the three overhead cost centres: administration, cleaning and pharmacy. (Note that this simplified, hypothetical hospital does not even have a kitchen.)
>
> The first column of Table A2 shows the total cost for each line item, including contributions from government, donors and elsewhere. The remaining columns show how this total cost is attributed to different cost centres. In some cases, an item is assigned to only one cost centre (e.g. cleaner's wages and cleaning supplies to "cleaning"). In other cases, items are attributed to several cost centres (some staff work on more than one ward, for instance). Also, some drugs are shipped direct to wards while most are shipped to the pharmacy.
>
> From Table A2, we see that the three wards incur 44% of the total costs. More than half of the total costs cannot be directly linked to a specific final cost centre, a proportion similar to that in many real hospital studies. The indirect costs must now be allocated using accounting rules (see page 17 and Box 4).

spent with each patient. This was supplemented by interviews with patients. The study authors found that physicians worked only 12% of the time for which they were paid. This is an example of how the process of cost analysis can generate important information, even without computing unit costs. (The information they gained was that the hospital was paying for labour it did not obtain.)

Comparison of approaches

The direct measurement approach has the advantage of giving direct information about the sources of inefficiency, where other approaches merely identify the cost centre to which expenditures should be assigned. The disadvantage of the direct measurement approach is the high cost of implementing it, at least in the way defined by Lewis and colleagues. Analysts may want to consider a more limited implementation, perhaps in the second phase of a hospital cost study after getting other systems working. The simplest method is to examine duty rosters for staff (if available), and allocate their time and associated salaries and fringe benefits accordingly.

Excluded activities

At some hospitals, certain activities generate costs which should be excluded from the unit cost computation. There are several possible reasons for such exclusion.

The prime example is teaching. Suppose one wishes to compare unit costs between some hospitals which do a lot of teaching and others which do not. The teaching hospitals will naturally appear to have higher costs, even if they provide patient care very efficiently. In this situation, it is desirable to identify and exclude teaching costs as far as possible. This may in part be done using job rosters which identify how many hours were spent teaching. However, teaching and patient care often occur simultaneously. Robertson and colleagues developed an approach to this in their Colombia study, which tracked physicians with time-and-motion methods. When care was being provided by a resident, the resident's time was charged to patient care while the supervisor's time was charged to teaching. When the resident and physician-supervisor conferred after seeing a patient, the time of both was charged to teaching.

Sometimes the central government operates some directly controlled programmes on the hospital premises (e.g. immunization campaigns). If these programmes are not under the hospital's control, it would be unreasonable to include them in the hospital's unit costs.

In both cases, the excluded activities should be treated as final cost centres, in the sense that overheads will be allocated to them and they will not be reallocated to other centres. However, unit costs will not normally be computed for them (unless one is particularly interested and can identify outputs to measure).

Drugs

Drugs usually account for a substantial share of hospital resources, so the way their costs are treated in an analysis is important. To compute a unit cost per prescription, one will definitely need to create a separate cost centre for drugs (e.g. "pharmacy"). If drugs are not to be treated as an output, two approaches are possible, namely:

— create a separate "pharmacy" cost centre but allocate its costs to final cost centres during the step-down process;

— assign drug costs to the cost centres (intermediate and final) before the step-down process.

Each approach has different advantages. The first approach is simpler, in that pharmacy costs will eventually be allocated on the basis of a single statistic (e.g. each ward's share of prescriptions written). The second approach has value if better information is available. For instance, if there is data on the value of each department's drug purchases, the currency amounts could be assigned to each department at this stage. However, there is also a managerial issue to consider: the pharmacy is usually a separate hospital department run by a manager or responsible person who should be able to track (and account for) use of the resources provided. The pharmacy manager will be better able to manage resources if the pharmacy is treated as a separate cost centre. In addition, identifying the pharmacy as a separate cost centre in all hospitals would

help regional and national managers to monitor and compare the relative performance of pharmacy departments in different hospitals. Therefore, this is the
preferred option, barring exceptional circumstances.

Allocating all costs to final cost centres

The next step is to reallocate all indirect costs to the final cost centres.
In this way, the unit cost will include overhead costs incurred in producing an
admission, day or visit, and not just direct costs. Indirect costs will include all
costs that could not be allocated directly to final cost centres at an earlier stage.
In some hospitals, indirect costs will comprise only services such as administration and laundry. In others, intermediate services such as pharmacy and
radiology may also need allocating at this point, with little or no information
about how much of their workload was generated by each of the medical
departments.

Allocation basis

Where each department's use of an indirect cost centre is unknown, one
must devise some rule to allocate the indirect costs across departments. The
rule is called an "allocation basis" and is intended to reflect whatever factors
determine each department's use of the indirect (i.e. overhead and intermediate) cost centre. These factors may differ depending on the centre. For
example, most studies allocate laundry costs between wards on the basis of the
percentage distribution of total patient-days in each ward, since patients who
stay longer use more laundry services. On the other hand, cleaning services are
often allocated according to each department's floor area, since the more spacious departments cost more to clean. (Of course, this may involve measuring
the floor area of each department if such information is not readily available
from sources such as building plans.)

If one knows a hospital well, one may be able to devise an allocation basis
which predicts costs accurately, even if it has not been used elsewhere. For
example, Weaver et al., the authors of the Niger study, decided that the number
of air-conditioning units would be a good predictor of water and electricity
costs, so they used that basis to allocate utility costs across wards (i.e. percentage distribution of air-conditioning units). They also learned that patients
in private wards were served better food, so that it would be incorrect to allocate kitchen cost simply based on the number of bed-days. Instead, they used
a weighting scheme in which one day in a private room was equivalent to several
days in the general ward.

Table 3 presents a summary of the bases for allocating various types of
overhead costs in previous studies (in those cases where methods were
described). For some services, a clear consensus is apparent, as in the use of
inpatient-days to allocate laundry. For others, there is more variation, with four
different methods being used to allocate maintenance. The large number of

empty cells (denoted by dashes) results from the very different ways cost centres were defined across these studies (e.g. electricity and water appear separately in some studies, but are combined as "utilities" in other studies).

Allocation using direct cost

A more rough-and-ready approach is to allocate all indirect costs on the basis of a department's percentage share of direct costs. This approach is discussed in Appendix 2; it is recommended only when other data are not available for allocating direct costs.

Step-down sequence

The order in which centres are allocated may affect final results and therefore deserves some consideration. Step-down analysis basically assumes that resource flows are in one direction, and that one can therefore make use of this in choosing the step-down sequence. Table 4 illustrates this by showing resource flows between overhead cost centres at a hypothetical hospital. The first row shows that the administration cost centre serves all others, so it should be allocated first. The next two rows show that the cleaning cost centre serves the pharmacy but does not receive drugs in return. The cleaning cost centre should therefore be allocated before the pharmacy cost centre. The order of the remaining rows does not matter since they will not be allocated (they are final output centres).

It may be a help to draw up a similar grid for overhead cost centres at one's own hospital. (It is not essential to include the final cost centres since their costs will not be allocated anyway, but it may be useful to include them because this will help to make clear which are the "receiving" departments.) Notice the shaded cells in Table 4 (below the diagonal of cells with dashes) which have no Xs in them. If the same area on a hospital grid has many Xs, they should be reduced by swapping rows (i.e. changing the order of the departments in the column and row headings). Xs below the diagonal introduce inaccuracy into the step-down process because one is forced to ignore some resource flows where the receiving department would already have had all its costs allocated. It is possible that even after swapping rows some Xs will remain below the diagonal. This is because, in reality, most hospitals do have some two-way resource flows (e.g. the administrative cost centre receives services from cleaning when its offices are cleaned). This is an unavoidable source of inaccuracy in simple step-down analysis, but it is probably less important than the more basic issues of cost measurement. (If necessary, techniques to handle two-way flows can be found in accounting texts such as Berman & Weeks, 1974.)

Table 5 presents the cost centres used in the Lesotho study, in reverse order. Allocation started with "all other administration" (no. 29) and finished with pharmacy (no. 11).

Table 3. Bases used for allocating overhead cost centres to intermediate and patient care cost centres (overview of prior studies by cost centre)

Study	Laundry	Kitchen (food)	Maintenance	Domestic	Transport	Cleaning	Administration	Utilities	Water	Electricity	Phone	Fuel	Security
Algeria	P	P	P	P	–	–	P	–	–	–	–	–	–
Bhutan (I)	–	D	–	–	A	–	PC	–	–	–	–	–	–
Bhutan (II)	–	–	F	–	A	–	P	–	–	–	–	–	F
Dominica	F	D	F	F	–	–	PC	–	–	–	–	–	–
Dominican Republic	A	D	F	–	–	F	DC	–	–	–	–	–	–
Ecuador	A	D/P	P	–	–	P	P	–	–	–	–	–	–
Egypt (II)	A	NS	DC	–	DC	–	–	–	–	–	T	–	DC
Gambia	D	D	F	–	DC	–	P	–	F	F	–	–	–
Jamaica	D	D	DC	DC	DC	DC	DC	DC	–	–	–	–	–
Lesotho	D	PC	PC	–	PC	–	PC	–	–	–	–	–	PC
Malawi	D	D	F	F	A	–	DC	–	–	–	–	–	–
Montserrat	–	D	F	F	–	–	PC	–	–	–	–	–	–
Niger	D	–	–	–	–	–	P	–	AC	AC	P	P	–
Papua New Guinea	D	D	DC	–	–	F	DC	–	–	–	–	–	–
Russian Federation	D	D	F	–	DC	F	P	–	–	–	–	–	–
Sierra Leone	D	D	F	–	–	–	DC	–	–	–	–	–	F
St Lucia	D	D	F	F	–	–	DC	–	–	–	P	P	–
Tuvalu	NS	NS	NS	NS	NS	NS	PC	NS	NS	NS	P	P	NS

A = estimated actual use
AC = air-conditioning units
B = beds
D = days of care
DC = direct cost
F = floor area

P = personnel numbers
PC = personnel cost
T = telephones
NS = not specified
— = not identified as a separate cost centre

Table 4. Resource flows in a hypothetical hospital

Department providing service	Department receiving service		
	Administration	Cleaning	Pharmacy
Administration	------	X	X
Cleaning		------	X
Pharmacy			------

Note: X denotes the flow of resources from the department providing the services to the department receiving them.

In some studies, the authors choose this point to separate inpatient and outpatient costs at certain cost centres. For example, some make the assumption that it costs three times as much to perform an inpatient surgical procedure as to perform an outpatient one. This allows them to allocate costs to inpatient or outpatient at the operating theatre cost centre.

Since inpatient and outpatient care are measured in different units (days versus visits), they should be costed separately. However, the inpatient/outpatient distinction should be made earlier in the step-down process by defining inpatient and outpatient surgery as separate cost centres. This allows the analyst to use information about how specific overhead items are used differently for inpatient and outpatient care. For example, outpatients may generate very few costs for kitchen and laundry but a disproportionately high share of costs for drugs. These differences should be tracked by cost centre rather than by using an across-the-board rule of thumb at the last stage. (Of course, the rule of thumb may be the only option if there is no better information available.)

Allocation of ancillary services

The allocation of costs of ancillary services is an important step, as they represent a substantial proportion of hospital costs. For X-ray and laboratory, most analysts try to estimate actual use. In the Papua New Guinea study, however, the number of admissions proved to be a good approximation (John Snow Inc., 1990).

Estimation of actual use involves gathering data on each department's share of utilization at the ancillary cost centre during a sample period. If one assumes that the sample period is typical of the whole year, one can then apply the proportion from the sample to the full year's data. For example, if during the sample period the surgical ward used 20% of total X-rays performed by the radiology department, one can assume it also used 20% of the annual X-ray volume.

There are two main ways to obtain the sample data needed for this approach. One is retrospective: review of past records kept by the ancillary

Table 5.   List of cost centres in the Lesotho study

A. Direct patient care
 1. Adult medical/surgical wards
 2. Theatre
 3. Obstetric wards
 4. Paediatric wards
 5. Satellite clinics
 6. Public health
 7. Dental
 8. Casualty
 9. Clinics
10. Nursing

B. Ancillary clinical services
11. Pharmacy
12. Laboratory and blood bank
13. Radiology
14. Physiotherapy
15. Orthopaedic workshop

C. Support services
16. Sterile supply
17. Maintenance
18. Security
19. Food service
20. Laundry
21. Portering
22. Transport
23. Mortuary

D. Administration
24. Medical records
25. Accounts
26. Personnel
27. Stores
28. Registry
29. All other administration

Source: Puglisi R, Bicknell W (1990). *Functional expenditure analysis: final report for Queen Elizabeth II Hospital, Maseru, Lesotho.* Boston, MA, Health Policy Institute, Boston University.

department, for one or more months. For example, the Papua New Guinea study found that the local hospital's radiology and laboratory departments kept logbooks for recording which departments had ordered each test. To avoid processing a whole year's logbooks, the authors sampled a 15-day period at each hospital and assumed that it would be representative of the whole year.

Another way to obtain sample data is to ask staff at the ancillary cost centre to track utilization by department over a short period of time. This approach has been used in the Dominican Republic (Lewis, 1990; 1995) and Jamaica (Kutzin, 1989). Typically, hospital staff in the X-ray, physiotherapy and laboratory cost centres are surveyed about the source of patients seen during one week (inpatient, outpatient) and the number and type (e.g. basic, special) of examinations performed. This information is then used to allocate ancillary costs to inpatient and outpatient care.

If no data can be obtained, interviews with staff may provide an approximate idea of utilization patterns. For example, in Kutzin's Jamaica study the national laboratory did not record its supplies to individual hospitals but laboratory staff were able to estimate rough shares for each hospital.

Concern with these approaches arises if an ancillary department produces various outputs of differing value and some departments are more likely to use the higher-cost outputs. For example, suppose that the medical ward uses more complex laboratory tests than the obstetric ward. In this case, the medical ward's share of laboratory tests will understate its true share of cost.

Various studies have dealt with this by assigning a "relative value" to each type of test, before computing departments' shares of volume. In some cases, there may be information in logbooks or ledgers about the relative value of different outputs. For example, some hospitals in francophone countries assign a "B-value" to each ancillary test, indicating its relative complexity (on a scale from 4 to 80). This value has been used to adjust for relative costliness of tests in studies of Algeria (Djelloul) and Niger (Wong, 1989).

Table 6 provides a comparison of how frequently these various methods were used in some of the studies reviewed. It may be noted that many studies used one basis to allocate ancillary costs to inpatient or outpatient care, and a different basis to allocate inpatient costs to wards or departments.

Box 4 and Table A3 continue the example by applying step-down cost analysis to the hypothetical hospital analysed in earlier boxes.

The step-down analysis for the hypothetical example is simpler than will be encountered in real applications. Consequently, a real-life step-down analysis is reproduced from the St Lucia study as Tables 7 and 8. Amounts are in Eastern Caribbean dollars (EC$), where EC$ 2.3 equals US$ 1. Table 7 shows the step-down analysis itself (slightly adapted from the original study), starting with direct cost figures for 11 indirect and 15 direct cost centres. (In this study, the ancillary departments were not allocated but were treated as final cost centres.) The second column shows each department's share of direct expense other than administration, and those shares are used to allocate the administration cost (EC$ 696 931) across the other cost centres. The process continues across subsequent pages until all indirect cost centres have been allocated. Table 8 then computes unit costs for the direct cost centres, using service units provided and the fully allocated cost from the step-down analysis.

This more realistic example yields several additional insights. First, if the step-down process is done by hand, there is some possibility of rounding errors. For example, the exact share of maintenance in non-administrative direct cost is 4.89214% (computed as 376 622 ÷ (8 395 428 − 696 931)). Using this share, one would allocate US$ 34 094.91 of the administrative cost to maintenance. However, if one had rounded the share to 5%, the amount allocated to main-

---

Box 4. Cost allocation in the worked example

Table A3 shows a simplified step-down allocation for the hypothetical hospital X. The first column shows the direct cost for each of the six cost centres, which was obtained earlier (Table A2). The first overhead cost centre to be reallocated is administration since it services all the other centres. The costs of administration are allocated to each of the other centres based on their share of the remaining direct cost (which is US$ 72000 after subtracting the direct cost of administration from the total cost). For example, the cleaning cost centre accounts for 15% of this remaining cost and is therefore allocated 15% of US$ 28000, which is US$ 4278. When this US$ 4278 is combined with the US$ 11000 in direct costs at the cleaning cost centre, this centre now has costs of US$ 15278. The other cost centres are each assigned a share of the administrative cost in the same fashion, proceeding down the same columns.

The next centre to be reallocated is cleaning. The fifth column shows that US$ 15278 in costs are to be reallocated from cleaning. These costs are allocated to each remaining department in proportion to its floor space. Since the pharmacy occupies 10% of the hospital's floor space, it is allocated 10% of US$ 15278, which is US$ 1528. Note that no costs are allocated to administration since it preceded cleaning in the step-down sequence.

The final reallocation is that of pharmacy. The only remaining cost centres are the three patient care wards. Pharmacy costs are allocated according to each ward's share of the value of direct drug shipments (recalling that some drugs were shipped direct to the wards). The medical ward has the highest proportion of such shipments and is assigned a correspondingly high share of the costs at the pharmacy cost centre.

The final column of Table A3 depicts the total of fully allocated costs at each ward at the end of the step-down process. Note that the total costs add up to US$100000; all the hospital's costs have been attributed to the three wards. Costs are highest for the medical ward, which also had the highest total direct cost. The next stage will show how costs compare to utilization in each ward.

---

tenance would be US$ 34846.55. This latter figure is 2.2% higher than the earlier, more exact allocation. The error will then be carried forward to subsequent stages. As far as possible, therefore, one should avoid rounding figures during the step-down process.

Costs not allocated to patient care

Although the aim is to allocate most of the hospital's costs to final output centres, some costs may not be relevant to production of admissions or days. For example, several studies computed the costs of teaching medical students or nurses but did not allocate those costs to any of the final cost centres for patient care. The idea is that resources used for teaching were not "necessary" for the production of medical care, so they should be excluded from its cost.

Table 6. Bases used for allocating ancillary cost centres to output centres (overview of prior studies by cost centre)

Study	Laboratory	Pharmacy	X-ray	Medical records	Operating theatre	Physiotherapy
Dominican Republic	A	A	A	AD	N	—
Ecuador	N	M	N	—	—	N
Egypt (II)	E/AD	M	AD	—	S	N
Gambia	E/AD	M	E/AD	AD	A	—
Jamaica	A/D	D	A/D	AD	S/A	A/D
Lesotho	E/D	E/D	E/D	D	N	E/D
Malawi	AD	A	M	—	S	—
Niger	M	A	M	—	—	—
Papua New Guinea	A	D	A	—	S	D
Sierra Leone	N	N	N	A	N	N
St Lucia	N	A	N	AD	N	N
Tuvalu	M	M	M	—	—	—

A = estimated actual use from sample
AD = admissions and/or outpatient visits
D = days of care and/or outpatient visits
E = estimates by employees
M = measured use over the study period

N = not allocated (final cost centre)
NS = not specified
S = number of surgeries
— = not identified as a separate cost centre

Note: Two-item cells (e.g. E/AD) denote two-stage allocation, with the first item (e.g. E) denoting the basis for allocating to either inpatient or outpatient, and the second item (e.g. AD) denoting the basis for deciding which inpatient service to allocate to.

However, exclusion of these costs is equivalent to creating a separate final cost centre for teaching (or whatever the other excluded activities are). Eventually, one may wish to have output measures for these other final cost centres too — in order, for instance, to find out whether productive resources are being allocated reasonably to teaching or to patient care.

Computing the unit cost for each cost centre

At this point the total costs that were incurred at each of the final cost centres are known. What is the output of each centre in days, discharges, laboratory tests and so on? Finding out requires utilization data to be incorporated into the analysis.

In reality, utilization data have already been used by this stage (e.g. to allocate laundry costs across wards in proportion to bed-days). However, this is the stage at which any problems with the utilization data become particularly important because they directly alter the unit costs.

Several studies encountered problems with utilization data. In some cases, the number of admissions seemed accurate but admission and discharge dates had not been carefully recorded, causing inaccurate measurement of bed-days.

Table 7 (Part 1). Step-down allocation, Victoria Hospital, St Lucia

Departments	Direct expense	Administration		Maintenance	
		Allocation statistic Direct expense	Allocation of expense	Allocation statistic Square feet	Allocation of expense
	EC$	%	EC$	%	EC$
Indirect departments					
Administration	696 931	[a]100.0	[a]696 931		
Maintenance	376 622	4.9	34 095	[a]100.0	[a]410 717
Domestic	299 774	3.9	27 138	0.2	821
Hospital stores	33 560	0.4	3 038	1.3	5 339
Pharmacy	89 991	1.2	8 147	1.1	4 518
Nursing administration	124 238	1.6	11 247	1.2	4 929
Laundry	141 776	1.8	12 835	6.2	25 464
Seamstress	139 174	1.8	12 599	0.2	821
Catering/kitchen	363 787	4.7	32 933	1.3	5 339
Medical records	71 235	0.9	6 449	1.9	7 804
Handymen	134 256	1.7	12 154	0.0	0
Subtotals	2 471 344	23.0	160 634	13.4	55 036
Direct service departments					
Maternity ward	596 511	7.7	54 001	4.7	19 304
Gynaecology ward	323 662	4.2	29 301	2.6	10 679
Baron (private) wing	216 956	2.8	19 641	4.8	19 714
Medical wards	738 291	9.6	66 836	11.2	46 000
Surgical wards	659 103	8.6	59 667	7.1	29 161
Paediatric ward	368 720	4.8	33 380	6.0	24 643
Ophthalmology ward	193 207	2.5	17 491	2.5	10 268
Operating theatre	1 181 195	15.3	106 931	7.9	32 447
Laboratory	489 830	6.4	44 343	2.4	9 857
Radiology	315 032	4.1	28 519	2.8	11 500
Physiotherapy	42 244	0.5	3 824	0.8	3 286
Mortuary	42 077	0.5	3 809	0.8	3 286
Casualty (with clinics)	622 010	8.1	56 309	5.4	22 179
Medical clinic	17 978	0.2	1 628	0.5	2 054
Psychiatric clinic	10 781	0.1	976	0.3	1 232
Subtotals	5 817 597	75.6	526 657	59.8	245 609
Other departments					
Nurses' home	106 487	1.4	9 640	20.4	83 786
Central medical stores (space only)	0			6.4	26 286
Subtotals	106 487	1.4	9 640	26.8	110 072
Totals	8 395 428	100.0	696 931	100.0	410 717

[a] Amount to be allocated, not included in total.

Table 7 (Part 2). Step-down allocation, Victoria Hospital, St Lucia (continued)

Departments	Domestic		Hospital stores		Pharmacy	
	Allocation statistic	Allocation of expense	Allocation statistic	Allocation of expense	Allocation statistic	Allocation of expense
	Square feet		Direct expense		Direct expense	
	%	EC$	%	EC$	%	EC$
Indirect departments						
Administration						
Maintenance						
Domestic	ª100.0	ª327 733	ª100.0	ª45 870	ª100.0	106 307
Hospital stores	1.2	3 933				
Pharmacy	1.1	3 605	0.1	46		
Nursing administration	1.3	4 261	0.1	46		
Laundry	6.1	19 992	5.2	2 385		
Seamstress	0.2	655	9.3	4 266		
Catering/kitchen	1.3	4 261	22.8	10 458		
Medical records	1.9	6 227	0.4	183		
Handymen						
Subtotals	13.1	42 933	37.9	17 385	0.0	0
Direct service departments						
Maternity ward	4.7	15 403	6.1	2 798	16.0	17 009
Gynaecology ward	2.7	8 849	1.8	826	10.9	11 587
Baron (private) wing	4.8	15 731	1.0	459	4.0	4 252
Medical wards	11.3	37 034	5.0	2 294	18.2	19 348
Surgical wards	7.1	23 269	4.3	1 972	15.8	16 796
Paediatric ward	6.0	19 664	1.6	734	9.1	9 674
Ophthalmology ward	2.5	8 193	1.0	459	4.0	4 252
Operating theatre	7.9	25 891	14.3	6 559	8.9	9 461
Laboratory	2.4	7 866	10.8	4 954		0
Radiology	2.8	9 177	10.9	5 000		0
Physiotherapy	0.8	2 622	0.1	46		0
Mortuary	0.8	2 622	0.1	46		0
Casualty (with clinics)	5.5	18 025	0.9	413	12.5	13 288
Medical clinic	0.5	1 639	0.0	0	0.5	532
Psychiatric clinic	0.3	983	0.0	0	0.1	106
Subtotals	60.1	196 968	57.9	26 559	100.0	106 307
Other departments						
Nurses' home	20.4	66 858	4.2	1 927	0.0	0
Central medical stores (space only)	6.4	20 975	0.0	0	0.0	0
Subtotals	26.8	87 833	4.2	1 927	0.0	0
Totals	100.0	327 733	100.0	45 870	100.0	106 307

ª Amount to be allocated, not included in total.

Table 7 (Part 3). Step-down allocation, Victoria Hospital, St Lucia (continued)

Departments	Nursing		Laundry		Seamstress	
	Allocation statistic	Allocation of expense	Allocation statistic	Allocation of expense	Allocation statistic	Allocation of expense
	Nursing staff		Patient days		Nurse staffing	
	%	EC$	%	EC$	%	EC$
Indirect departments						
Administration						
Maintenance						
Domestic						
Hospital stores						
Pharmacy						
Nursing administration	[a]100.0	[a]144 720				
Laundry			[a]100.0	202 452		
Seamstress					[a]100.0	[a]157 516
Catering/kitchen						
Medical records						
Handymen						
Direct service departments						
Maternity ward	13.9	20 116	17.2	34 822	13.9	21 895
Gynaecology ward	6.6	9 552	11.0	22 270	6.6	10 396
Baron (private) wing	7.3	10 565	5.5	11 135	7.3	11 499
Medical wards	16.5	23 879	24.9	50 411	16.5	25 990
Surgical wards	16.8	24 313	22.6	45 754	16.8	26 463
Paediatric ward	10.2	14 761	15.3	30 975	10.2	16 067
Ophthalmology ward	6.6	9 552	3.5	7 086	6.6	10 396
Operating theatre	13.1	18 958		0	13.1	20 635
Laboratory	0.0	0		0	0.0	0
Radiology	0.0	0		0	0.0	0
Physiotherapy	0.0	0		0	0.0	0
Mortuary	0.0	0		0	0.0	0
Casualty (with clinics)	8.7	12 591		0	8.7	13 704
Medical clinic	0.2	289		0	0.2	315
Psychiatric clinic	0.1	145		0	0.1	158
Subtotals	100.0	144 720	100.0	202 452	100.0	157 516
Other departments						
Nurses' home	0.0	0	0.0	0	0.0	0
Central medical stores (space only)	0.0	0	0.0	0	0.0	0
Totals	100.0	144 720	100.0	202 452	100.0	157 516

[a] Amount to be allocated, not included in total.

27

Table 7 (Part 4). Step-down allocation, Victoria Hospital, St Lucia (continued)

Departments	Catering/kitchen		Medical records		Handymen		Total (allocated cost)
	Allocation statistic Nursing staff	Allocation of expense	Allocation statistic Patient days	Allocation of expense	Allocation statistic Nurse staffing	Allocation of expense	
	%	EC$	%	EC$	%	EC$	EC$
Indirect departments							
Administration							
Maintenance							
Domestic							
Hospital stores							
Pharmacy							
Nursing							
Laundry							
Seamstress							
Catering/kitchen	[a]100.0	[a]416 778					
Medical records			[a]100.0	[a]91 898			
Handymen					[a]100.0	[a]146 410	
Direct service departments							**Total cost**
Maternity ward	17.2	71 686	12.6	11 579	17.2	25 183	890 306
Gynaecology ward	11.0	45 846	4.7	4 319	11.0	16 105	493 390
Baron (private) wing	5.5	22 923	1.4	1 287	5.5	8 053	342 213
Medical wards	24.9	103 778	5.5	5 054	24.9	36 456	1 155 370
Surgical wards	22.6	94 192	6.6	6 065	22.6	33 089	1 019 845
Paediatric ward	15.3	63 767	8.7	7 995	15.3	22 401	612 781
Ophthalmology ward	3.5	14 587	1.4	1 287	3.5	5 124	281 901
Operating theatre							1 402 078
Laboratory							556 850
Radiology							369 228
Physiotherapy							52 022
Mortuary							51 840
Casualty (with clinics)			56.6	52 014			810 533
Medical clinic			2.2	2 022			26 456
Psychiatric clinic			0.3	276			14 657
Subtotals	100.0	416 778	100.0	91 898	100.0	146 410	8 079 470
Other departments							
Nurses' home							268 697
Central medical stores							47 261
Subtotals	0.0	0	0.0	0	0.0	0	315 958
Totals	100.0	416 778	100.0	91 898	100.0	146 410	8 395 428

[a] Amount to be allocated, not included in total.

Table 8. Unit cost calculation, Victoria Hospital, St Lucia

Department	Total cost	Units of service	Units	Unit cost
	ECS			ECS
Maternity ward	890306	Day	9866	90
Gynaecology ward	493390	Day	6295	78
Baron (private) wing	342213	Day	3148	109
Medical wards	1155370	Day	14228	81
Surgical wards	1019845	Day	12946	79
Paediatric ward	612781	Day	8745	70
Ophthalmology ward	281901	Day	2009	140
Operating theatre	1402078	Operation	2642	531
Laboratory	556850	Test	60823	9
Radiology	369228	X-ray	8964	41
Physiotherapy	52022	Treatment	5561	9
Casualty (with clinics)	810533	Visit	34052	24
Medical clinic	26456	Visit	1327	20

Source: Russell et al., 1988 (slightly modified).

Box 5. Final computation of unit cost in the worked example

Table A4 presents the final computation of unit cost for the hypothetical Hospital X. The fully allocated costs for each ward, from Table A3, are now divided by the days of care on each ward. Although the medical ward had higher total costs, it also had many more days of care than the surgical ward (500 compared with 300). Unit costs are actually lower on the medical ward than on the surgical ward, at US$ 76 compared to US$ 96 per day.

As discussed, in some contexts it may be desirable to present intermediate results (i.e. those obtained before allocation of ancillaries). Table A5 shows what the unit costs look like if pharmacy is treated as a separate patient cost centre that does not allocate its costs. In this case, the total cost numbers in Table A5 come from column 7 of Table A3 (i.e. the cost figures after allocating administration and cleaning, but before allocating pharmacy). The results show a similar pattern to that in Table A4, with surgery having a substantially higher cost per day than either medicine or maternity. However, with pharmacy costs kept out, it is also possible to compute a separate cost per prescription, which is US$ 5 in this hypothetical case.

Correct measurement of bed-days requires that staff count how many beds are occupied in every ward every 24 hours at the same time of day. The authors of the Lesotho study recommended that this should be done at midnight. A recent report on a Zambian hospital gives details on one way to conduct a bed census (Buve & Foster, 1995).

Once the utilization data are obtained, the unit cost can be computed (as in Table 8 above). For each of the final cost centres, the fully allocated cost should be divided by the units of service (see Box 5).

Reporting results

At this point it is important to remind oneself what items are and are not included in the unit costs that have been calculated. For example, the unit cost does not include drugs and X-rays unless these services were specifically allocated to the final patient cost centres during step 5.

Similarly, if one is not reporting outputs for certain final cost centres (e.g. teaching, public health clinic), then it is worth saying so in a footnote. Otherwise, readers of the report may assume these centres' costs have been allocated to the services for which unit costs are reported.

Chapter 2

Using cost data to improve management of a hospital

This chapter discusses uses of cost data within a hospital; it therefore aims to show departmental and programme managers and hospital administrators how costing can help improve their performance. The chapter focuses on two levels of decision-making:

— cost centre level (cost centre or department management);
— hospital level (financial and hospital management).

At each level of decision-making, uses of cost data will be drawn from seven categories of tasks:

— budgeting;
— variance assessment;
— profitability;
— efficiency improvement with regard to both allocative and technical efficiency (i.e. identifying areas of waste that can be corrected, pricing policy, and other health financing and policy concerns such as the projection of future costs);
— expansion or contraction of services;
— contracting outside services or producing in-house;
— enhancing cost–effectiveness of programmes and hospitals at the national level (e.g. comparing alternative approaches such as ambulatory with inpatient surgery to control a given medical condition).

Costs can be classified in different ways according to the type of decision facing the manager.

If the concern is how to allocate total hospital cost between different departments, a distinction must be made between:

— direct cost, which can be directly assigned to a particular cost centre (e.g. surgical supplies to the surgery cost centre);
— indirect cost, which cannot be directly assigned (e.g. electricity bills, which are not usually itemized by the amount of electricity used by each department).

31

If the concern is how to vary input use in response to changing demand, then a distinction must be made between:

— variable costs, which change with the quantity of patient care (such as visits or patient-days);
— fixed costs, which do not change when the quantity of patient care changes.

For example, if patient-days drop by 10%, one would expect lower costs of meals and laundry, implying that they are variable inputs. However, in the short term, the fall in patient-days may have no effect on total wage costs, since the hospital cannot dismiss workers without notice. Over the short term, wages are a fixed cost. Over a longer period (e.g. one year), adjustments may become possible, making wages a variable cost in the long term. Thus, the longer the time period, the larger the portion of cost that may become variable.

The first section of this chapter discusses the various uses of cost data at the level of the cost centre which tend to be in the areas of budgeting, variance assessment, profitability, efficiency (allocative and technical), expansion or contraction of services, and deciding whether to contract outside vendors/providers as opposed to using in-house staff to provide services. Examples in this section focus on analysis of cost variance at departmental level and the usefulness of cost analysis when considering whether to purchase contractual services or use in-house staff.

The second section applies cost analysis at the hospital level for budget development and monitoring, determining profitability status, pricing services, and identifying waste and technical inefficiencies. Other issues facing managers of large tertiary hospitals and smaller district hospitals are also discussed. Examples in this section focus on issues of profitability and budgeting.

Cost data at cost centre or department level

By creating cost centres, assigning costs to them, and allocating them to final patient service departments, hospital directors and financial officers learn the quantity of resources used to produce each hospital service. Departmental directors and cost centre managers also learn the amount of resources they are responsible for managing. There are other benefits to having this information: improved management, more financial accountability among departmental managers, and benchmarks developed for measuring departmental performance over time (e.g. number of meals served, cost of a radiological examination, total personnel cost of eye care and so on). Perhaps the foremost reason for examining levels and determinants of costs is that it provides useful insight into the relative efficiency of hospital operations.

At the level of the cost centre or department, the major uses of cost analysis are the calculation of cost variances and unit costs as measures of efficiency.

Cost variances are differences of an actual dollar[1] amount from a standard amount (benchmark). These are the clues that signal that a potential problem exists and suggest a possible cause. Common examples of such variances are:

— all variances that exceed an absolute dollar size (e.g. US$ 500 or 15 000 rupees;

— all variances that exceed budgeted or standard values by some fixed percentage (e.g. 10%);

— all variances that have been unfavourable for a defined period (e.g. 3 months);

— some combination of the above.

Actual cut-off or criteria values (or "rules") in the above examples are highly dependent on management judgement and experience. A variance of US$ 1000 (or, for example, 30 000 rupees) may be considered normal in some circumstances and abnormal in others. In each case, the objective of cost variance analysis is to assess why actual costs differ either from budgeted values or from actual values of a prior period.

Budget variance

The historical approach to budget variance allows a hospital director to assign responsibility to managers of cost centres and to hold them responsible for the budget performance of their respective departments. In turn, variance assessments will allow the manager of each department to compare the department's actual costs against budgeted figures. The budget variance is calculated as:

budget variance = budgeted cost − actual cost.

Thus, positive numbers are favourable and negative numbers are unfavourable (or are considered deficits).

Intertemporal variances

In general, the primary reason for a cost change at the departmental level between two time periods is a function of three factors:

— changes in input prices;

— changes in input productivity (efficiency);

— changes in departmental volume.

The following variances can be calculated to compute the effects of these factors:

— *input prices:* price variance = (present price − old price) × present quantity;

---

[1] The word "dollar" is used as a simplification. Any currency could be substituted.

— *input efficiency:* efficiency variance = (present quantity − expected quantity at old productivity) × old price;

— *volume changes:* volume variance = (present volume − old volume) × old cost per unit.

As shown in the following example, these formulas can be applied in analysing cost changes at departmental level.

Example 1: Departmental analysis of cost variance

Lakshmi Hospital in India is a fictitious 325-bed referral hospital that provides patient care, teaching and research. It is modelled after actual experiences of certain hospitals in India. In 1996, bed occupancy for the entire hospital was 75% but increased to 85% during 1997. As might be expected, Lakshmi's laundry service department was affected by this bed occupancy change.

From cost accounting studies done in 1996 and 1997, the hospital administrator suspects that unit costs in the laundry department have gone up. Perhaps she has compared the total costs in the laundry department with the total inpatient-days and sees that laundry costs per day have increased. She knows that the increase in unit cost could have been caused by an increase in bed occupancy, as well as by increases in prices and wages (i.e. inflation), or by a drop in the productivity (input efficiency) of the laundry department. She can disaggregate the direct costs in the laundry cost centre into personnel costs and supply costs but needs more detailed information in order to determine the source of the unit cost increase. Therefore, she asks the manager of the laundry department to provide the needed details. The laundry manager is able to track records of the total volume of laundry done in each year (in kilograms), the total number of boxes of soap used each year, the price per box of soap used, and the number of workers employed each year at the hospital laundry. Using this information together with information from the study on salary (plus fringe benefits) costs in the laundry cost centre, the laundry manager assembles the basic information needed in Table 9.

As shown in Table 9, the department uses only two inputs — soap and labour. (Note that to avoid rounding errors, several decimal places were retained. Fixed costs for space are discussed below.) Box 6 gives the resulting variances.

On the basis of these calculations, Table 10 summarizes the factors that created cost changes in the laundry department.

In the Lakshmi Hospital example, the increased volume (or output) was the largest source (51.7%) of the total change in cost, with a decline in labour efficiency being the smallest source of change (0.2%). However, all inputs combined (price and efficency of labour, price and quality of soap) contributed to 48.3% of total cost changes in comparison with 51.7% for volume output.

34

Table 9. Laundry service at Lakshmi Hospital

Item	1996	1997
Total recurrent costs of laundry cost centre (rupees)	2016000	3315000
Total labour costs	216000	435000
Total soap costs	1800000	2880000
Kg of laundry	90000	120000
Recurrent cost per kg of laundry (in rupees)	22.400	27.625
Boxes of soap	1200	1600
Soap boxes per kg of laundry (boxes of soap/kg of laundry)	0.01333	0.01333
Price (in rupees) per box of soap	1500	1800
Number of staff (average per year)	7.5	10
Hours worked (staff × 8 × 365)	21600	29000
Hours per kg of laundry (hours worked/kg of laundry)	0.240	0.242
Wage rate (in rupees) per hour	10	15

Box 6. *Variance components for Lakshmi Hospital*

Price variances
Soap = (1800 rupees − 1500 rupees) × 1600 boxes of soap
        = 480000 rupees (unfavourable)
Labour = (15 rupees − 10 rupees) × 29000 hours worked
        = 145000 rupees (unfavourable)

Efficiency variances
Soap = 1600 boxes of soap − [0.01333 soap boxes per kg of laundry
        × 120000 kg of laundry] × 1500 rupees
    = 0 rupees
Labour = 29000 productive hours worked − [0.24 productive hours per kg of
            laundry × 120000 kg of laundry] × 10 rupees
        = 2000 rupees (unfavourable)

Volume variances
Volume variances = (120000 kg of laundry produced in 1997 − 90000 kg of laundry
                produced in 1996) × 22.400 rupees
        = 672000 rupees (favourable)

The key managerial issue is to identify the extent and causes of a change in input efficiency. The results of the analysis show that there was virtually no change in input efficiency. Thus, the laundry manager can reasonably claim that the increase in unit and total costs was not the fault of the laundry department but rather the result of general inflation and an increase in service volume.

Table 10. Lakshmi Hospital laundry department: causes of cost changes, 1996–1997

Cause	Rupees	% change
Increase in soap prices	480 000	37.0
Increase in wages	145 000	11.1
Change in soap quality	0	0.0
Decline in labour efficiency	2 000	0.2
Increase in volume	672 000	51.7
Total change in cost	1 299 000	100.0

Box 7. Input cost variances of components

Input 1: Soap

Soap = (1600 boxes of soap × 1800 rupees per box) − [(1200 boxes × 1500 rupees per box) × (120 000 kg of laundry ÷ 90 000 kg of laundry)]

= 2 880 000 rupees − (1 800 000 rupees × 1.33333)

= 480 000 rupees (total cost variance for soap)

Input 2: Labour

Labour = (29 000 productive hours worked × 15 rupees per hour) − [(21 600 hours × 10 rupees per hour) × (120 000 kg of laundry ÷ 90 000 kg of laundry)]

= 435 000 rupees − (216 000 rupees × 1.33333)

= 147 000 rupees (total cost variance for labour)

Input cost variance

Example 2 below shows how input prices and efficiency can be combined in input costs. If there are several inputs, it may be impractical to measure the quantities used for each. In that case, it is possible to divide cost changes between inputs (which combine price and efficiency of all inputs) and outputs. In the following formula, input cost variance can be calculated for all inputs combined, for a group of inputs, or for each input separately:

input cost variance = present input cost − [old input costs × (present volume ÷ old volume)].

Example 2: Calculating input cost at departmental level

Using the laundry department as an example, input cost variances of component inputs are given in Box 7.

Box 8 presents the combined input costs in this example.

The system of cost variance analysis described above is a useful framework for analysing the sources of changes in departmental costs. It is recommended that this approach be limited to examining major supply categories;

Box 8. Combined input costs

Combined cost variance $= 3\,315\,000 - [2\,016\,000 \times (120\,000\,kg + 90\,000\,kg)]$
$$= 3\,315\,000 \text{ rupees} - 2\,688\,000 \text{ rupees}$$
$$= 627\,000 \text{ rupees}$$

We can verify that this sum is correct by showing that it equals the sum of the components of the two inputs.

Input 1 (soap) cost variance + input 2 (labour) cost variance = combined input cost variance

$480\,000$ rupees + $147\,000$ rupees = $627\,000$ rupees

---

there may be little use in calculating price and efficiency variances for each of a hundred or more supply items. For smaller areas of supply or material costs (e.g. pencils, sheets of paper, boxes of paper clips), a simple change in cost per unit of departmental output may be just as informative as detailed price and efficiency variances.

Contracting services versus in-house production

Analysis of unit costs also allows managers to compare the economic advantages of contracting services with those of in-house staff. Private contractors may have better access to capital for new vehicles and equipment, better access to cash for buying parts, flexibility in hiring staff with the necessary skills, and flexibility to adjust staffing to the workload by season, day of week and time of day.

The measure of unit costs for an internal (or in-house) ancillary or support service can be compared with the cost of purchasing the same service from a private contractor. In addition to cost, numerous aspects of "quality" complicate the examination of contracting options. Quality includes not only the service itself (how well and how promptly it is carried out), but also other administrative, political and personnel dimensions. Important elements are the employment security of workers in the support service and the nature of the infrastructure provided. Workers may oppose the contract option, particularly if their job security is not guaranteed. Yet private contractors may be reluctant to manage a public service at an advantageous price if they have no control over the workforce. A compromise is usually possible that gives hiring preference to the former public-service workers.

Purchasing of support services under contract is becoming more common in developing countries. For instance, the Ministry of Health in Sierra Leone purchases catering services under contract at all provincial hospitals. Spanish-town and other hospitals in Jamaica contract out for support services such as portering and catering, with managerial support from the United States Agency for International Development (USAID).

Both long-term and short-term costs, which take account of equipment and use of space as well as operating costs, need to be considered. Example 3, again based on the laundry service at Lakshmi Hospital, illustrates these trade-offs. The manager distinguishes variable costs (which vary with the amount of laundry) from fixed costs (which do not vary).

Example 3: Deciding whether to replace laundry equipment or contract out

In 1997, Lakshmi Hospital's laundry manager determined that all of the hospital's current laundry machinery would no longer be serviceable in 1998. New equipment, which is produced domestically, would cost US$ 63700 (1 911 000 rupees). He now faces the decision whether to replace the equipment or close the laundry and contract the work out to a private supplier who has adequate capacity to handle the hospital's 132 000 kg of laundry. Assuming 3% inflation for domestic equipment and methods (Box 6), the annual depreciation of the new equipment would be US$ 10 000 (300 000 rupees) per year. The fixed cost per kg of laundry for the new equipment would be 2.2727 rupees, based on 132 000 kg of laundry per year. Added to the existing fixed cost (for space), the overall fixed cost would be 6.25 rupees per kg. After requesting bids from local vendors, the best quote was a price of 32 rupees per kg of laundry for three years. The resulting cost comparison (in rupees) is as follows:

	Contract services	Use in-house staff
Variable cost per kg	32.0	30.3875
Fixed cost per kg	included	6.2500
Total cost per kg	32.0	36.6375

Based on the above cost comparisons, it is recommended that the laundry department contract the work out to the local vendor provided that:

— the quality of services is maintained or increased;
— current in-house laundry personnel can be hired by the private contractor and/or employed elsewhere in the hospital;
— other costs (such as inventory or replacements) do not increase;
— current space can be used by the hospital for other purposes.

If these conditions are satisfied, the hospital will save 4.6375 rupees per kg (calculated as 36.6375 less 32.0) or 612 000 rupees (US$ 20 400) per year.

Cost data at hospital level

Cost variance analysis

Cost variance analysis is also of great importance to the hospital director or administrator. He or she is interested in analysing the institution's overall performance, or in analysing how changes in one department affect another. The unit of analysis at the hospital level is a single cost centre or a combination of cost centres within a particular department. In our fictitious example, the occupancy of Lakshmi Hospital's inpatient clinical units rose from 75% in 1996 to 85% in 1997. Again considering the laundry department, the hospital director may be interested in knowing to what extent both intensity of services and "pure volume" contributed to the 51.7% volume increase from 1996 to 1997.

Example 4: Analysis of cost variance at the hospital level

For the hospital director, the next step is to determine whether the 51.7% volume variance was due to intensity of services (e.g. increase in kg of laundry per patient-day) or change in volume due to change in overall service (e.g. increase in total patient-days). These two factors are computed as follows:

intensity = (change in volume due to intensity difference)
      × old cost per unit
pure volume = (change in volume due to change in overall service)
      × old cost per unit

According to previous information, 1.01159 kg of laundry were provided per patient-day in 1996 and 1.19011 kg per patient-day in 1997.

Box 9 presents the volume variances in this example.

Budgeting

Hospitals can use cost information to establish rates (fee levels) and comply with both internal and external reporting requirements, to determine whether departments are operating within budget, to construct a budget for a department (or new initiative), and to allocate budgets between departments or cost centres.

As shown in Box 10, variance analysis can be applied in constructing the next year's budget for a department. To do this, the management of Lakshmi Hospital identifies those elements of cost that are presumed to be fixed and those that are presumed to be variable. Fixed costs do not change with respect to changes in volume whereas variable costs do change. We assume that variable costs change in direct proportion to changes in output or volume. That is, if output increases by 10%, these variable costs may also increase by 10% (a constant cost increment per unit of output). In the next example, output in the laundry department is expected to increase by 10% due to a 10% increase in bed occupancy (from 85% to 93.5%). Variable cost is expected to increase due to both 10% annual inflation and the output increase. Fixed cost is expected to increase by only 5% as only some components (e.g. utilities and maintenance) rise in cost while others (e.g. depreciation) remain constant.

Box 9. Volume variances

Fiscal year 1996: 325 beds × 75% occupancy rate × 365 days = 88 969 total patient-days. 90 000 kg of laundry ÷ 88 969 total patient-days = 1.01159 kg of laundry per patient-day in 1996.

Fiscal year 1997: 325 beds × 85% occupancy rate × 365 days = 100 831 total patient-days. 120 000 kg of laundry ÷ 100 831 total patient-days = 1.19011 kg of laundry per patient-day in 1997.

Based on the above information, the two volume variances are:

intensity variance = [(1.19011 − 1.01159) × 88 969 total patient-days in 1996] × 22.4 rupees
= 355 775 rupees

pure volume = 1.19011 × (100 831 total patient-days in 1997 − 88 969 total patient-days in 1996) × 22.4 rupees
= 316 225 rupees

We can verify that the two volume variances are correct by showing that they equal the total volume variance of 672 000 rupees:

volume variance = intensity variance + pure volume variance
= 355 775 rupees + 316 225 rupees
= 672 000 rupees

Box 10. Constructing the 1998 budget for the laundry department of Lakshmi Hospital

The cost equation may be represented as follows:
total 1998 budget = (fixed cost + variable costs)

1998 variable costs = (120 000 kg of laundry × 1.10 output growth factor) × (27.625 × 1.10 inflation factor)

= 132 000 kg of laundry × 30.3875 rupees per kg of laundry
= 4 011 150 rupees

1998 fixed costs = 500 000 rupees × 1.05 inflation factor = 525 000 rupees

1998 total budget = 4 011 150 rupees + 525 000 = 4 536 150 rupees

Note: 27.625 is the 1997 unit cost.

Example 5: 1998 budget variance for the laundry department of Lakshmi Hospital

As part of the annual financial review process, the administrator of the hospital examines the laundry department's 1998 budget in relation to actual experience. Table 11 presents the relevant data. Overall, the laundry department has a favourable budget variance of 66 150 rupees.

Table 11.   Budget data for Lakshmi Hospital

Item	1998 actual	1998 budget	Variance	Interpretation
Quantities:				
Laundry (kg)	125 000	132 000	7 000	(unfavourable)
Costs:				
Variable costs (rupees)	3 945 000	4 011 150	66 150	(favourable)
Fixed costs (rupees)	525 000	525 000	0	(neutral)
Total costs (rupees)	4 470 000	4 536 150	66 150	(favourable)[a]

[a] *Note*: The interpretation is favourable because of underspending relative to the budgeted level. However, the hospital manager could be dissatisfied since the underspending is due primarily to volume being less than anticipated.

Fiscal solvency

Fiscally autonomous hospitals are those in which the hospital management (the administration and/or the hospital board) has both the authority and the responsibility to maintain the financial viability of the hospital. These hospitals include private for-profit hospitals (increasingly common in major cities), public hospitals operated by independent authorities (such as major teaching hospitals), and private non-profit hospitals (such as those operated by religious or other nongovernmental organizations). Administrators of autonomous hospitals can use cost and revenue data to assess the overall "breakevenness" of the hospital (i.e. the extent to which revenues were equal to total expenses for a particular fiscal year).

"Breakevenness" is also relevant for revenue-producing departments like food services for visitors and families or clinical departments like internal medicine, surgery, or physical medicine and rehabilitation. The favourable difference between total revenues and total expenses (or costs) is called a profit or surplus. The unfavourable variance is called a deficit or loss. Determining and attaining a level of profitability that is both acceptable and sufficient is not easy. If profits are too low, quality of care can be seriously impaired because of an insufficiency of resource support, both personnel and capital. In the long run, the viability of the institution may be threatened because of an inadequate capital base that will ultimately restrict ability to expand clinical or ancillary services, to pay for increasing costs such as personnel, or to reconstruct an old building. If profits are too high, the community may feel exploited by its hospital.

Example 6: Determining the fiscal solvency of Lakshmi Hospital

Table 12 presents the data for assessing the "breakevenness" of the hypothetical teaching hospital. This hospital is paid by patients, insurers and governments according to the services that it provides.

The most commonly cited measure of profitability is the operating margin ratio:

$$\frac{\text{net operating income}}{\text{total operating revenues}}$$

For Lakshmi Hospital, the value of this ratio in 1996 is:

$3\,250\,000 \div 54\,518\,000 = 0.0596$

The higher the value of the ratio, the better the hospital's financial condition. A simple way to understand this ratio is to think of it as a measure of profit retained per dollar of sales. For example, in 1996 Lakshmi Hospital retained 6 cents of every revenue dollar (or 6 rupees per 100 rupees of revenue) as profit. Given this relatively low operating margin, Lakshmi Hospital may need to examine its rate structure, increase its bed occupancy rate, and examine its cost structure to find costs that could be contained.

Table 12. Lakshmi Hospital: statement of revenue and expenses for the year ended 31 December 1996 (approximately 30 rupees equal one US dollar)

Item	Rupees
Patient service revenues[a]	61824000
Allowances and uncollectable accounts	7956000
Net patient service revenue	53868000
Other operating revenue[b]	650000
Total operating revenue	54518000
Operating expenses	
Nursing services	12306000
Medical and clinical services	10907000
General services[c]	8285000
Administrative services	7683000
Education and research	5285000
Depreciation	3888000
Interest	2806000
Total operating expenses[d]	51160000
Net operating income	3250000
Non-operating revenue[e]	360000
Excess of revenues over expenses	3610000

[a] Patient user fees, insurance payments, and government reimbursements. This amount is equivalent to 695 rupees (US$ 23.17) per patient-day.
[b] Visitor meals and gift shop.
[c] Support services (e.g. laundry and housekeeping).
[d] This amount is equivalent to 575 rupees (US$ 19.16) per patient-day.
[e] Donations.

Hospital revenues

The revenue generated by a hospital, expressed as a proportion of its costs, is the product of three factors: the fee level (average fee as a proportion of average unit cost), the proportion of services for which a charge is made (not exempted), and the collection efficiency (proportion of fees owed which are actually collected and remitted to the hospital's account). Generally, only a proportion of patients are actually charged the set fee, with the remainder being exempted due to poverty or other defined categories (e.g. schoolchildren, disabled war veterans).

The fee level and the proportion of patients required to pay are policy variables set by the hospital or the ministry of health. The need for a high degree of acceptability and a high degree of affordability for the service argues for setting these percentages low. The demand for treatment of illnesses which are less severe is generally more sensitive to price ("price elastic", in economic terms) than the demand for treatment of more severe illnesses. This factor argues for more subsidy for outpatient care. Also, the demand for treatments that are expensive (i.e. requiring a high share of the household's available cash) are more sensitive to price than those which are less expensive. This factor may sometimes work in the opposite direction as an argument for more subsidy for inpatient care. Considerations of cost–effectiveness favour the principle of subsidizing services that make a substantial impact on health in relation to their cost (these include childhood vaccinations, vitamin A supplementation, treatment of respiratory infections, and treatment of tuberculosis). This last factor is a measure of administrative capacity. The efficiency of fee collection is greatest when hospital systems are designed to facilitate enforcement of fee payments. For example, the flow of patients may be designed so patients must pass first by a registration window and obtain a receipt prior to obtaining care, a drug, or a laboratory test. Such procedures are easier to implement for elective care, when patients or family members can be expected to bring funds to the hospital, than for emergency services.

The three factors are summarized in Table 13. The "current situation" represents the authors' impression of fee collections in government hospitals in Bangladesh and Zimbabwe, where this manual was discussed in workshops. The fee level is currently low overall because fees for inpatient services and drugs generally cover only a small share of the costs involved, and these costs represent the majority of the operating costs of the hospitals. The proportion of patients paying fees is also low because of broadly defined policies of exemption. As hospitals do not retain the fees they collect, they have every reason to be generous in interpreting the need for an exemption. Finally, the collection factor reflects the absence of specific programmes to enhance collection.

When a government subsidizes the hospital sector, it is useful for the administrator of each hospital to determine the net public subsidy his or her institution receives. The subsidy is calculated as:

Table 13. Factors explaining rate of cost recovery

Factor	Interpretation	Current situation %	High fee %	Moderate fee %
Fee	Full fee for paying patients as proportion of unit costs	20	100	85
Proportion paying	Proportion of patients exempted from fees	50	50	50
Collection	Proportion of fees not exempted actually collected	40	60	70
Recovery	Proportion of costs recovered	4	30	30

net subsidy = hospital costs – hospital revenues.

Hospital administrators can use the level of subsidy to help guide decisions over which they have control, such as certain expenditures, application of policies about exemptions from fees, and efforts towards fee collection. They can also use this measure in developing or evaluating proposals about their hospital for regional and national government officials. For example, they could argue prospectively that an investment in additional capital or operating costs could increase revenues and thereby reduce the subsidy. They could also negotiate an understanding to share any reduction in subsidy between the hospital and government as a whole. Retrospectively, they could request that all or part of any reduction in subsidy be reinvested in the hospital to ensure the viability of ongoing efforts to limit the net subsidy.

In Jamaica, where a comparable collection rate previously existed, efforts of the Health Sector Initiatives Program substantially increased revenues. Hospitals were given the liquidity, and flexibility of spending their revenues rose. Collectors were trained, building modifications were made if necessary to create a cashier's window, and additional positions were created to ensure that cashiers were on duty during evenings and weekends in addition to normal hours.

The "high fee" scenario in Table 13 shows what would happen if nominal prices were set with no subsidies (i.e. 100% of costs). With only a moderate proportion of patients asked to pay (50%) and a moderate level of collections (60%), the overall level of cost recovery is 30%. By contrast, the same revenue is raised with a more moderate level of fees (15% lower on average) and the same level of exemptions (50%) but with better collections (70% enforcement). In some hospitals, "leakage" in collections occurs between the patient and the hospital accounts. Where the patient may pay an "informal" fee, it may be retained by a gatekeeper, personal attendant, aide, nurse or physician, or deposited in a location other than the official hospital accounts.

Chapter 3

Using cost data to improve management of a hospital system

T his chapter discusses cost analysis of a hospital system. It covers the simplest hospital system, the district or province, and the national level. At district level, managers may have the authority to set prices and allocate budgets to district health services in systems where such decisions are decentralized to district level. This chapter focuses on improving the referral system within the district and the appropriate use of different providers of services.

At national level, the chapter suggests ways to identify inefficiencies in different but similar types of hospitals nationally or within a specified geographical area (i.e. province, state or region). It focuses on improving the referral system between hospitals and on the appropriate use of different providers of services. It also covers the cost–effectiveness of programmes, and whether the hospital should provide high-level curative care or preventive primary care.

Estimating volumes and costs in a hospital system

In some hospitals, data are so limited that costs cannot be analysed with the techniques described in Chapter 2. None the less, it is still possible to draw some conclusions even if one has only aggregate cost data and limited service or activity data. This section discusses what analyses can usefully be performed in such situations, and the limitations of these analyses.

Projections from very limited data

The most limited situation is one in which only two very limited types of data are available for an individual hospital or a group of similar hospitals: the total operating costs and some measure(s) of size or activities. The preferred measure of size or activities is the number of services performed during a given period (such as the last year). A usable proxy, however, is the number of beds.

Shepard and Gonzales (1982) used this approximation to project the cost impact of a major expansion in hospitals in Honduras from 1980 to 1983. With data on the numbers of beds and recurrent costs for general public hospitals, they calculated that the annual operating cost per bed had grown at a 6.9% real annual rate from 1976 to 1980 because of increasing intensity of services

Table 14. Projecting costs of hospital services in Honduras (in US$ at 1980 value)

Item	Actual 1980	Projected 1983
Number of beds	3579	4490
Annual operating cost per bed (US$)	5708	6973
Total cost of hospital system (US$ million)	20.4	31.3
Projected real increase over 1980	n.a.	53%

n.a. = not available.

(or simply because of increasing budget allocations). They used this trend to project the future cost per bed. They multiplied it by the projected future number of beds (calculated by adding the number of beds under construction or planned to the existing bed capacity). As shown in Table 14, real costs were projected to rise by 53% in just three years. The increase would have represented more than the entire budget for ambulatory care in the country's health system.

To the consternation of financial officials, the results proved realistic. With the construction and planning processes well under way, the ministry of health and donors added the beds essentially as scheduled. Financial constraints delayed the opening of several hospitals, however, until years after they were completed.

Similar approaches could be applied to an individual hospital, or to various types of hospital systems, such as:

— all government district hospitals in a given region, or in the country as a whole;
— all provincial hospitals in the country;
— all multipurpose referral or teaching hospitals in a given region, or in the country as a whole;
— all specialized hospitals with a given purpose, such as mental health or tuberculosis.

Estimating costs from relative values

A more accurate approach is feasible if data are available on the volume of services produced (activities) for a hospital over a defined period (generally one year), as well as on the annual operating costs. This approach differs from that in Chapter 3, however, because it does not require operating costs to be assigned to individual departments or cost centres. Deriving unit costs from these data entails five steps.

• *Identify the output-producing centres.* As in Chapter 2, one must decide for which services unit costs will be computed. This depends primarily on the level of detail for which activity data are available. For most hospitals, data are available on at least the aggregate number of ambulatory visits and the aggregate number of inpatient bed-days per year. In this case, one can estimate total cost of inpatient versus outpatient care and the unit costs of a bed-day and ambulatory visit. In some cases, the number of bed-days is reported by clinical department or ward (e.g. medicine, surgery, maternity), in which case one can estimate the unit costs per bed-day by ward.

- *Define units of output.* For each patient care cost centre, one must define a unit of output. Within cost centres, the unit of output must be readily counted and reasonably uniform. In most cases, inpatient services are best expressed in terms of days, and ambulatory services in terms of visits. Inpatient admissions represent an alternative, though less uniform, measure. Costs will then be expressed per day or per visit. If data are available on admissions as well as patient-days, this will allow for a calculation of average length of stay. Average cost per admission could then be calculated by multiplying the estimate of average cost per day by the average length of stay.
- *Define the data period.* Data can be analysed on a per year, per quarter or other basis. It is crucial to make sure that the same time period applies to both the aggregate cost figure and the utilization data.
- *Identify the full costs of the facility.* Financial statements for the hospital may be a useful starting point although, as previously noted, they may understate cost. Where possible, one should try to add in costs of resources used by the hospital but paid for by others, such as donated items, drugs purchased by a central state agency, or employees' time paid for out of other budgets. (See pages 5–13 for a full discussion of how to develop complete cost data.)
- *Obtain external data on relative costliness of services.* To implement this approach, estimates of the relative costliness of different types of care are needed. Such estimates could be, for example, that one day of inpatient care costs three times as much as one outpatient visit, or that one surgical admission costs 10% more than the average inpatient admission. These data are called "external" because they have to come from outside the hospital. (If such data exist internally, one could probably use the techniques described in the previous chapter rather than those in this one.) Possible sources for these estimates could include:
  - other hospitals in the country for which step-down cost accounting studies (as described in Chapter 2) have been carried out;
  - the judgement of clinical experts or hospital staff on the relative amounts of resources used for the different services;
  - studies from other countries;
  - Table 15, which shows relative values for a variety of services. These relative values are derived from the review of those step-down studies for which unit costs were available. (Owing to the small numbers, separate relative values by type of hospital are not pro-

Table 15. Relative values for estimating costs by service[a]

Service	Unit	Mean	Relative value Range (low-high)	Number of observations
All inpatient care[b]	day	1.00	—	19
Medical with intensive care unit	day	1.28	0.67–3.54	8
Medical only	day	0.81	0.67–0.96	5
Intensive care unit only	day	2.65	1.39–4.79	5
Surgical with operating room	day	1.26	1.10–1.50	7
Surgical only	day	0.77	0.56–1.01	6
Operating room only	operation	4.92	0.24–8.16	7
Obstetrics and gynaecology	day	1.00	0.50–1.33	10
Obstetrics only	day	1.21	0.81–2.08	7
Gynaecology only	day	0.99	0.84–1.21	3
Paediatrics	day	0.84	0.49–1.39	15
Outpatient	visit	0.32	0.12–0.60	14

[a] A department's relative value is the ratio of its cost per day (or per visit for outpatient care) to the overall average inpatient cost per day.
[b] The relative value for this service was set as equal to one.

vided. However, more useful information will be generated if estimates are used from similar hospitals, e.g. hospitals in the same country, or same level of hospital.)

Example 1: Relative values with costs by inpatient ward

Table 16 shows how this calculation would work for a hypothetical hospital that provides only inpatient care. We begin by identifying what we want to calculate and what we already know prior to manipulating the data. In this case, we want to calculate the average cost per day in the medical, surgical and maternity wards. What we know is total hospital expenditure (US$ 100 000), and total inpatient-days in each of the three wards. Thus, in order to make the simplified unit cost calculation using the relative value approach, we need only to identify the relative cost of a day in each ward.

The steps in this example were as follows:

- *Patient care cost centres.* As before, we distinguished between medical, surgical and maternity (but not pharmacy). The results are therefore comparable to those in Table A4 (see page 67).
- *Unit of analysis.* We chose the day as the unit of analysis, because estimates of relative costliness are more readily available on a per day basis than per discharge.
- *Time period.* Although monthly utilization data are available, the financial data are annual so we calculated unit cost on an annual basis.
- *Relative values.* We took the ones from the analysis presented in Table 15.

Table 16. Unit cost calculation from relative values for a hypothetical hospital

Ward	Reported items			Calculated items			
	Total cost (US$)	Inpatient-days	Relative value	Relative value units	% of relative value units	Cost of each service (US$)	Cost per inpatient-day (US$)
Medical (no ICU[a])		500	0.81	405	32.8	32 847	66
Surgical with operating room		300	1.26	378	30.7	30 657	102
Obstetrics and gynaecology		450	1.00	450	36.5	36 496	81
All inpatient	100 000	1250	1.00	1233	100.0	100 000	80

[a] Intensive care unit.

- *Calculations.* The first column reports the total cost to be apportioned. The second column repeats the inpatient-days by ward, from Table A4. The third column introduces the relative value weights from other studies, as presented in Table 15. Use of these weights implies that we assume that, compared to the average inpatient-day, a surgical day is 26% more costly and a medical day is 19% less costly. The fourth column uses these weights to convert days into relative value units (RVUs). It may be noted that although the medical ward provides more days than maternity, it provides fewer RVUs because each medical day has a lower relative value. The fifth column computes each ward's share of total RVUs. The sixth column applies that share to the total hospital cost of US$ 100 000 (from Table A1). For example, the surgical ward has 30.7% of the RVUs, so we assume it is responsible for 30.7% of the hospital's cost, or around US$ 30 657. Finally, each ward's total cost is divided by the inpatient-days (first column) to obtain the unit cost by ward. The surgical ward has a cost of US$ 102 per day, compared with US$ 81 per day for the maternity ward and US$ 66 per day for the medical ward.

How can these figures be used? We can use them to compare surgical costs across hospitals, or to see whether it would be cheaper to transfer some surgical patients elsewhere. We cannot use the results to conclude that surgery days are costlier than obstetrics and gynaecology days because this was an assumption we made and not something we learned from doing the analysis.

Comparison to step-down results

In the present case, we can return to the results of step-down analysis in Chapter 1 and see whether the "relative value" approach gives different results. (This would not be possible if one were unable to do step-down analysis in the first place due to poor data.) How different are the results?

Comparing Tables A4 and 16, we see that the relative value method understates unit costs by 14% for medical care and overstates unit cost for obstetrics and gynaecology (maternity) by 10%. The unit cost for surgery is the same for both approaches. (The overall cost per day is the same in both tables, since we have changed only the way total costs are allocated across wards and not the amount of total cost or days of care.)

From the comparison, we can conclude that our rules of thumb were somewhat inaccurate for two of this hospital's wards. Using the findings from our step-down analysis, the correct rules of thumb would have specified that a medical day costs only 1% less than the average inpatient-day, not 19% less. Also, maternity days are less costly than the overall inpatient average, not equally costly as specified by our rule of thumb.

Example of approach with costs by inpatient/outpatient visit

Table 17 provides another worked example, this time for a different hospital which knows only the total cost and the total number of inpatient-days and outpatient visits, but not the allocation of costs between inpatient and outpatient settings. This hospital can still estimate separate unit costs for inpatient and outpatient care by applying the relative values from Table 15 to its utilization data.

The first two columns show that this hospital incurred a cost of US$ 10 000 and provided 100 inpatient-days and 1200 outpatient visits during the period studied. The third column gives the relative value weights from Table 15, which assume that one inpatient-day costs the same as about three outpatient visits. Column 4 uses the weights to convert days and visits into RVUs, and column 5 shows the share of RVUs provided in each setting. Since inpatient care accounts for 20.66% of RVUs, we assume it also accounts for

Table 17. Unit cost calculation from relative values: inpatient versus outpatient

Service	Total cost (US$)	Units	Relative value	RVUs	% of RVUs	Total cost (US$)	Unit cost (US$)
Inpatient		100 days	1.00	100	21	2066	20.66/day
Outpatient		1200 visits	0.32	384	79	7934	6.61/visit
Total	10000	—	—	484	100	10000	—

RVU = relative value unit.

20.66% of total cost, that is US$ 2066. This gives an inpatient cost per day of US$ 20.66. Similarly, the outpatient cost per visit is US$ 6.61.

The above example shows that the relative value approach can be applied even if different departments use different units. Even though the inpatient department provides days and the outpatient department provides visits, the two can be compared by converting dissimilar units to a common standard (the relative value).

Strengths and limitations of these approaches

The strength of the approaches described is their simplicity. The requirements in data are few; the analytical computations are easily done with a calculator. It is easy to explain the derivations. Also, results are likely to be less susceptible to misunderstanding when only approximate data are available.

The limitation of these approaches is the potential for inaccuracy if the estimates used are not appropriate for the hospital being studied. One reason for this is that relative values are likely to differ by type of hospital. For example, it may be that an inpatient-day in a teaching hospital is really five times costlier than an outpatient visit. If managers do not know this and use the 1:3 ratio from Table 17, they may understate inpatient unit costs (and overstate outpatient costs).

Allocation of a budget between hospitals

Bed-day equivalents provide a useful statistic to allocate a central budget equitably between public hospitals. If this statistic were the only one used, each hospital would receive a budget proportional to its share of total bed-day equivalents. That is, if a hospital generated 10% of the country's bed-day equivalents in the latest year with full data, it would be awarded 10% of the country's hospital budget next year. This statistic is one of the terms in the formula used by the Zimbabwe Ministry of Health to allocate funds to its central hospitals.

While not perfect, this system has several advantages. It is more objective and rational than allocations based on past budgets and political influence. It rewards productivity and efficiency, so each hospital receives the same budget per inpatient-day and per outpatient visit. By contrast, budgets based on historical costs perpetuate, and may even encourage, overspending and inefficiency.

Limitations of a system based on bed-day equivalents are its exclusion of several important factors and its possible perverse incentives. A system based solely on bed-day equivalents would fail to account for needs for preventive and promotive services (which are not measured by inpatient and outpatient services), for differences in the sophistication of services, for other factors affecting the costs of services (e.g. distance and scale), for varying abilities of hospitals to raise revenue (based on the capacity to pay of the

51

populations they serve), and for the time and central support required for a hospital to adjust to a different budget (i.e. to transfer personnel in or out, trim costs responsibly, or use additional funds productively). Perverse incentives can arise because such a system would reward provider-induced utilization (i.e. excessive admissions, lengths of stay, or follow-up visits to boost activity statistics).

These limitations can be addressed by incorporating other factors in the allocation formula and by using a blended formula based on a combination of bed-day equivalents and historic budgets. The Zimbabwe Ministry of Health has addressed many of these concerns by using 13 parameters (including bed-day equivalents) in its allocations of resources. Other factors include population (a proxy for overall service needs), area (a proxy for distance between facilities), numbers of health facilities and of rural health clinics (measures of scale), total beds, number of vehicles, laboratory units (all measures of sophistication), staff salaries and allowances (measures of past budgets), and outpatient attendances, patient-days, and occupied beds (all additional measures of volume of activities). Each hospital's allocation is a weighted average of its share of the national total with regard to each of these factors. While the Zimbabwe system does not explicitly incorporate the relative income of catchment populations in its formula, this could be included in a final manual adjustment allowed by the system.

Improving hospital efficiency

Overall efficiency

The manager of a hospital system should calculate the unit costs of final outputs for each of the hospitals in the system and should compare the results for the same unit of service in hospitals of the same type (e.g. district, provincial, referral). For example, costs per patient-day and per outpatient visit can be compared.

First, it is important to be careful in interpreting results for comparing efficiency across wards or hospitals. Although wards with a lower unit cost may be more efficient, it is also possible that they are treating healthier patients, or providing lower-quality care (e.g. inadequate provision of drugs). These explanations should be considered, even if one eventually decides that they do not apply in the case one is analysing. If several hospitals have comparable sources of referral and comparable reputations, then it is plausible that they treat a comparable mix of patients. If important, case mix could be quantified by tallying the proportion of patients with diagnoses classified as more serious or determining the proportion of patients referred from other institutions. Provision of drugs per case could be quantified by counting the number of essential drugs prescribed and furnished by the hospital and dividing by the total number of patients, or by determining the proportion of prescribed drugs that were dispensed through the hospital pharmacy.

For hospitals of comparable sophistication and quality, a low cost per patient-day is an indication of good efficiency, while a high cost per patient-day may suggest poor efficiency. A manager will first want to examine the data to rule out three spurious factors. First, if unit costs are excessively high in one hospital, resources may have been over-allocated to that hospital and under-allocated to another. For example, if two institutions share some important service, such as a pharmacy, but all or almost all of the cost is allocated to just one institution, then the costs of that institution would be inappropriately high while the costs of the other would be inordinately low. The manager should examine the unit costs of hospitals that might share services to see if they are inordinately low. If so, the manager should consider revising the basis of allocation of the shared resource to see if results change substantially.

Second, the share of resources allocated to a particular service may have been inappropriately high. For example, if a hospital's cost for an outpatient visit is high, perhaps an excessive share of personnel or pharmacy costs has been allocated to that service. To determine whether this spurious factor is responsible, the manager should examine possible reallocations of that resource. A service which represents a small share of a hospital's total costs is especially prone to errors in allocation. A small absolute difference in allocation will then make a big relative change in unit costs. For example, a manager may be unsure whether an emergency (casualty) ward represents 5% or 10% of hospital personnel. The total personnel costs, and thus the unit personnel costs, will be twice as high with a 10% allocation. For a large service, however, a 5% difference is much less crucial. The difference of 5% between, say, a 50% and a 55% share of personnel for medical/surgical inpatient stays would change unit costs by only one-tenth. If unit costs for a given hospital tend to be very high for some services and very low for others, it is possible that the basis of allocation is inappropriate. On the other hand, if a hospital's unit cost is consistently above average for different services, then that hospital is probably less efficient than the average.

Third, an especially low unit cost may indicate that important resources are not being counted, or an estimate for a resource is particularly high. Results from Connaught Hospital in Sierra Leone may indicate this kind of situation. Many drugs and supplies were not bought officially through the hospital pharmacy (which had limited stock), but were purchased by patients either through commercial pharmacies in the city or through semi-formal drug sales at the hospital pharmacy. Knowledge of how a hospital operates makes the situation clearer.

Once these spurious factors have been ruled out, it is instructive to examine the most efficient hospitals. Characteristics worth noting are: occupancy rate, staffing per bed, staffing per patient-day, and the proportion of staff who are doctors (including dentists and licensed pharmacists), other health

53

and management professionals (including nurses, technicians, therapists and administrators), and non-professionals (drivers, aides, housekeepers).

The standards of the most efficient hospital are often worth emulating.

Analysis of intermediate cost centres

Cost analysis involves the breakdown of total and unit costs by cost centres. Managers can judge the results against policy norms of how money ought to be spent, as well as against data on how money actually was spent at other times and in other hospitals.

For example, the Sierra Leone study (Ojo et al., 1995) reported that food for patients represented the majority of costs in the country's referral hospital. As food is a less essential part of the process of hospital treatment than professional advice and medicines, it does not deserve a larger share of hospital budgets. Thus, anomalous allocation of resources prompts an examination of why food costs are so high. Both data anomalies and real managerial characteristics need to be examined. In Sierra Leone, Ojo et al. (1995) reported that the cost of food (the equivalent of US$ 5 per patient per day) was based on an estimate of the value of food given by an international donor. Either the estimate was high, or the food provided was worth exceptionally high amounts.

Similarly, it is possible to compare the results of a specific cost centre in different hospitals. This can be done by examining the cost of this cost centre through three ratios: (1) overall costliness: costs per patient-day, (2) intensity: units of service per patient-day, and (3) unit costs: cost per unit of service. The first ratio measures the overall resources used by a cost centre, combining both utilization and costliness of that cost centre. The second ratio is derived by measuring the allocated units of service of an intermediate cost centre divided by the total units of service of the final cost centre. The third ratio is derived by dividing the total cost of the intermediate cost centre by its allocation statistic. The three ratios are related mathematically as (1) = (2) × (3). This relationship allows the consistency of the data to be verified. Box 11 shows how these concepts apply to the cleaning costs of the medical cost centre of the hypothetical Hospital X. Box 12 extends these calculations to all cost centres. Different officials are often responsible for the different ratios. While responsibility is shared for the cleaning cost per bed-day, the service intensity largely reflects choices in partitioning space between services, while the unit costs reflect the decisions of the person responsible for the cleaning service.

Refining the hospital's role in the health system

The unit of analysis at the health system level is all hospitals within a particular district, province or region, or the country as a whole.

Box 11. Interpretation of cost ratios for the cleaning service in hypothetical Hospital X

Table A3 shows that the cost of the cleaning cost centre allocated to the medical service was 3056 (based on cleaning supplies and the cleaner's salary). The text indicates that this cost centre was allocated on the basis of the floor area for direct care (the floor area for administration is not considered, since that cost centre has already been allocated). Suppose the total patient care floor area is $10000\,m^2$. Table A3 also shows that the medical cost centre accounts for 20% of the hospital's direct care floor area (i.e. $2000\,m^2$). Table A4 shows that this service has 500 units (patient-days). Thus, the first ratio (the cleaning cost per day) is 6.11 (calculated as $3056 \div 500$). The second ratio, the intensity of inputs, is the number of square metres per patient-day, or $2000\,m^2 \div 500$ patient-days, or $4\,m^2$ per patient-day. The third ratio (the unit costs of the cleaning service for the medical service) is the allocated cost (3056) divided by number of units (i.e. medical service floor area of $2000\,m^2$) giving a cost per square metre of 1.53 (calculated as $3056 \div 2000$). The consistency relationship is satisfied, subject to rounding (i.e. 6.11 is approximately equal to 1.53×4).

The calculations are:

Ratio 1	Ratio 2	Ratio 3
Cost/day =	$(m^2$ cleaned/day) $\times$	$(cost/m^2$ cleaned)
=	$(2000 \div 500)$ $\times$	$(3056 \div 2000)$
=	4 $\times$	1.53
≈ 6.11		

Box 12. Efficiency calculations for each service in Hospital X, and their interpretation

Comparable calculations can be made for each service, as shown below:

Service	Ratio 1 Cost/day	Ratio 2 Intensity	Ratio 3 Unit costs
Medicine	6.11	4.00	1.53
Surgery	15.28	10.00	1.53
Maternity	13.58	8.89	1.53

Results show that surgery has the highest cost per day and also the greatest intensity of floor area cleaned per patient-day. Maternity ranks second and medicine last. The unit costs are identical for all three services because they are based on assigned floor area. These results are generally consistent with the needs of each service for operating theatres (in surgery) and delivery rooms (in maternity), compared to beds alone in medicine. Comparing the results for each service in Hospital X to results for other hospitals provides important measures of efficiency.

Appropriate type of hospital

One of the principles of health planning is that patients should be treated in the least complex and least costly type of health facility that is adequate for their needs. This rule generally ensures that patients are treated more conveniently, at less cost to the family (because they save travel expenses), and often at lower cost to the health system (as lower-level facilities are thought to be less costly). Unit cost analysis allows the economic rationale behind this policy to be examined. For example, are tertiary hospitals really producing care more expensively than lower-level hospitals? If the tertiary hospitals have unit costs three times higher for the same services, should their fees also be three times higher?

Of course, cost is not our only concern. Important dimensions of quality must be examined. Quality entails not only the excellence of the staff, the depth of their training and the sophistication of their infrastructure; promptness and courtesy of service are also highly valued by patients. Nevertheless, there are potential economic gains from a more rigorous management of referral procedures.

Disease-specific costs

Among adults, the prevalence of HIV infection in developing countries in 1996 (1.5%) was 13 times higher than in industrialized countries (0.12%) (Mann & Tarantola, 1996). To better plan responses for prevention and control, both donors and national governments need data on current levels of health expenditures related to HIV/AIDS, as well as information on the allocation and sources of funds for this purpose. Hospital costs represent a critical component of overall costs. In a study sponsored by the World Bank, the European Commission and UNAIDS, Shepard (1996) selected five countries of varying economic levels for case studies. Only the one with the highest per capita gross domestic product, Brazil, had existing data on hospital expenditures for AIDS. These were derived from reimbursements through its government-run social security system.

For the other countries, several sources of data needed to be assembled. Côte d'Ivoire illustrates this process (Shepard, 1996). Estimates for Côte d'Ivoire were based on both objective data and Delphi estimates (i.e. judgements) by AIDS experts from government, voluntary hospitals and the field of traditional medicine (Koné et al., 1996). Table 18 shows the process used to reveal hospital costs. First, the overall number of AIDS patients in this country of 14.3 million persons was derived by taking the number of reported cases and expanding for under-reporting. Second, the experts classified the estimated annual number of new HIV/AIDS clinical cases (18 122) into five groups based on the expected type and amount of care that they typically received. Third, the length of stay and setting for each group was based on clinical data. Fourth, unit costs in each type of hospital were based on available unit cost studies,

Table 18. Cost of hospital care for HIV/AIDS patients in Côte d'Ivoire, 1995

Patient financing and location	Total number of cases	Days per patient	Cost per day[a]	Cost per patient[a]	Total days	Total cost[a]
Private coverage	906	34.0	52.5	1785	30804	1617210
Civil servants	1812	20.0	10.6	212	36240	384142
Other urban Abidjan	8699	16.3	15.0	245	141794	2126906
Other urban interior	3624	14.0	5.0	70	50736	253680
Rural	3081	5.0	5.0	25	15405	77025
Total or average[b]	18122	15.2	16.2	246	274979	4458965

[a] All monetary amounts are in thousands of CFA francs, where 1000 CFA francs equal US$ 2.00.
[b] This row represent totals for columns with heading beginning with "Total", and averages for other columns.

derived from step-down analyses or relative value approaches. For example, patients with private insurance coverage were estimated to receive care at private clinics, costing on average 52 500 CFA francs (equivalent to US$ 105) per day. At the other extreme, the hospitals used by rural patients (largely public district hospitals) cost 5000 CFA francs (US$ 10) per day. Finally, totals were calculated.

The overall average was 16 200 CFA francs (US$ 32.40). The 18 122 HIV/AIDS patients in Côte d'Ivoire received an estimated 274 979 bed-days of hospital care in 1995. The total cost of their hospital care was 4.46 billion CFA francs (US$ 8.9 million). Comparison with independent data on the hospital sector showed that HIV/AIDS patients represented about 21% of all hospital days and 19% of all hospital costs. Given that the country's seroprevalence is about 5%, these estimates were plausible.

By knowing the typical pattern of financing for each group of patients, the authors were able to estimate the overall financing of hospital care. Governments, which heavily subsidized public hospitals, provided 43% of costs; insurance (serving primarily civil servants and workers in large private-sector enterprises) financed 22% of costs; households (through user fees) supported 33%, and others (primarily donors) the remaining 3%.

These data permitted comparisons of actual expenditures and recommended allocations. Compared with other countries in the study, hospitals were both relatively costly and heavily used. Thus, hospitals consumed 48% of curative expenditures. Overall, curative care represented 92% of all HIV/AIDS expenditures in Côte d'Ivoire, compared with 58% in the five case studies overall. Côte d'Ivoire and other countries are using these data to refine their AIDS policies. In the short term, hospital costs can be reduced by providing care in less costly settings, such as ambulatory care or care in district hospitals, rather than in teaching hospitals. In the long term, more vigorous prevention programmes, such as those to detect and treat other sexually trans-mitted diseases, can help stem the increase in AIDS cases.

Cost–effectiveness analysis: disease control approaches

Cost analysis can help policy-makers compare alternative approaches to controlling a given disease. First, it can allow simple comparisons, such as ambulatory versus inpatient surgery. A Colombian study, for example, found that ambulatory surgery for repair of an uncomplicated hernia cost only one-quarter of what inpatient surgery cost (Shepard et al., 1993).

Cost analysis can also allow different approaches to disease control to be compared. For example, for two important health problems in many tropical countries, prevention is difficult. Respiratory infections are airborne. Dengue viruses are carried by mosquitoes that breed quickly, even when spraying has reduced their number. Cost–effectiveness analysis of control programmes for both diseases showed that, except for vaccination, case management was gen-erally the most cost-effective control procedure (Stansfield & Shepard, 1993; Shepard & Halstead, 1993). An analysis of hospital costs helped derive the costs of the case management approach.

Hospital financing: user fees

Cost analysis can be an important element in setting levels of user fees, although in practice fee-setting is also guided by other considerations. Cur-rently, hospital services in the public sector are heavily subsidized in almost every country. User fees commonly recover only one-tenth of hospital costs.

Governments can, and often should, continue to subsidize care at public hospitals. Nevertheless, the calculation of unit costs allows that subsidy to be allocated more rationally. Principles of social welfare policy indicate that sub-sidies should be granted under certain conditions. First, if the consumers of a service are poor, the subsidy is like an in-kind income transfer to them. Second, if the service is a merit good or has broad health benefits beyond the individ-ual patient, the government may want consumers to use it. Many primary care services, and especially immunization, fit this second category.

The above analysis suggests that there is little rationale for subsidizing amenity services that are consumed primarily by the well-off. On the contrary, amenity services should be priced to cover at least their own cost and, prefer-ably, to generate a surplus to subsidize the rest of the hospital. The most direct way of performing this analysis is to make the amenity service a separate cost centre for which the unit cost is calculated separately.

The St Lucia example in Tables 7 and 8 illustrates this process. Victoria Hospital had a private wing, called the Baron wing. Its daily cost was EC$ 109 per day. By contrast, the daily costs of the regular wards were EC$ 78 in gynae-cology, EC$ 79 in surgical, EC$ 81 in medical, EC$ 90 maternity and EC$ 82 overall (an average of these four adult wards, weighted by the number of bed-days in each). Thus, the daily cost of the amenity ward was 33% higher than that of the regular adult wards. A further analysis of the data in Table 7 shows that the higher costs of the private ward applied to both direct costs (29% higher) and indirect costs (39% higher). This example also illustrates the importance of using relevant statistics for allocating indirect costs in costing amenity services. The amenity ward represented 4.8% of the hospital's square footage, but only 2.8% of its direct expense or 1.4% of its patient-days. By contrast, the regular wards represented only 25.6% of the square feet, but 30.1% of the direct costs and 29.4% of the patient-days. As two categories of indirect costs (maintenance and domestic) were allocated on the basis of floor area, this procedure appropriately allocated extra costs to the private ward for its more spacious accommodation.

Principles of equity argue that the charge per day in the amenity ward should thus be at least EC$ 109 (US$ 47) per day. This charge could be made up of a combination of an admission fee, daily room and board charge, and itemized charges for drugs (to cover pharmacy) and medical supplies (to cover medical stores).

Hospital financing: insurance

A number of developing countries are considering, or are starting to implement, systems of national health insurance. For example, Colombia passed a health reform law in 1994. Trinidad and Tobago completed a major study, and Côte d'Ivoire is planning pilot programmes. Typically, these health insurance systems entail payment by the insurance to the provider of care (a hospital or doctor). Unit cost analysis allows an appropriate rate of payment to be developed.

Where countries allow multiple insurers to emerge, there is some risk that each insurer will try to pay less than its share of the hospital's overhead. This has been a problem in the United States, where some insurers have allegedly shifted costs to others by setting low payment rates. Measuring unit costs can help sort out these issues by distinguishing direct costs of an admission (to be paid by the insurer responsible) from overhead costs (to be prorated across insurers). In principle, the government could prevent cost-shifting by requiring every insurer to pay the unit cost of a discharge. In practice, this may be undesirable as hospitals may lose their incentive to restrain overhead costs (Ma, McGuire & McGuire, 1993).

References

Methodology of cost analysis

Barnum H, Kutzin J (1993). *Public hospitals in developing countries: resource use, cost, financing*. Baltimore, MD, Johns Hopkins University Press.

Berman HJ, Weeks L (1974). *Financial management of hospitals*. Ann Arbor, MI, Health Administration Press.

Creese A, Parker D, eds. (1994). *Cost analysis in primary health care: a training manual for programme managers*. Geneva, World Health Organization.

Hanson K, Gilson L (1996). *Cost, resource use and financing methodology for basic health services: a practical manual*, 2nd ed. New York, UNICEF (Bamako Initiative Technical Report Series, No. 34).

Over M (1991). *Economics for health sector analysis: concepts and cases*. Washington, DC, World Bank.

RAND Corporation (1992). *Unit cost analysis: a manual for facility administrators and policymakers (Working draft)*. Santa Monica, CA, RAND Corporation (Document WD-6282-MOH/RI).

Young DW (1984). *Financial control in health care: a managerial perspective*. Homewood, IL, Dow-Jones-Irwin.

Country studies

Bamako Initiative Management Unit (1994). *Cost, resource use and financing of district health services: a study of Otjiwarongo district, Namibia*. New York, UNICEF (Bamako Initiative Technical Report Series, No. 22).

Bijlmakers L, Chihanga S (1996). *District health service costs, resource adequacy and efficiency: a comparison of three districts*. New York/Harare, UNICEF/Zimbabwe Ministry of Child Health and Welfare.

Carrin G, Evlo K (1995). *A methodology for the calculation of health care costs and their recovery*. Geneva, World Health Organization (unpublished document WHO/ICO/MESD.2; available on request from Department of Health in Sustainable Development, World Health Organization, 1211 Geneva 27, Switzerland).

Djelloul B (no date). *Hôpital spécialisé en maladies infectieuses d'El-Kettar (Alger)*. Algiers, Ministère de la Santé et des Affaires Sociales.

Foley G et al. (1995). *Financial management and budgeting of health services at Connaught Hospital: a further analysis*. Geneva, World Health Organization, 1995 (unpublished document; available on request from Department of Health in Sustainable Development, World Health Organization, 1211 Geneva 27, Switzerland).

Gambia Ministry of Health/WHO (1995). *Cost analysis of the health care sector in the Gambia.* Geneva, World Health Organization (unpublished document; available on request from Department of Health in Sustainable Development, World Health Organization, 1211 Geneva 27, Switzerland).

Gill L (1994). *Hospital costing study: Princess Margaret Hospital.* Boston, MA, John Snow Inc. (Project report, No. 10).

Gill L, Percy A (1994). *Hospital costing study: Glendon Hospital — Montserrat.* Boston, MA, John Snow Inc. (Project report, No. 15).

Huff-Rousselle M (1992). *Dzongkhag costing study for Tashigang Dzongkhag.* Thimphu, Department of Health Services, Bhutan Ministry of Social Services.

Huff-Rousselle M (1992). *Financial study of Thimphu General Hospital: recurrent cost analysis and selected options for privatization and user fees.* Thimphu, Department of Health Services, Bhutan Ministry of Social Services.

John Snow Inc. (1990). *Papua New Guinea: health sector financing study project. Final report: Vol. II. Hospital cost study.* Boston, MA, John Snow Inc.

Kutzin J (1989). *Jamaican hospital restoration project: final report.* Bethesda, MD, Project HOPE.

LaForgia G, Balarezo M (1993). *Cost recovery in public sector hospitals in Ecuador.* Bethesda, MD, Abt Associates (Health Financing and Sustainability Technical Note, No. 28).

Lewis MA (1990). *Estimating public hospital costs by measuring resource use: a Dominican case.* Washington, DC, Urban Institute.

Lewis M et al. (1995). *Measuring public hospital costs: empirical evidence from the Dominican Republic.* Washington, DC, World Bank.

Mills AJ (1991). *The cost of the district hospital: a case study from Malawi.* Washington, DC, World Bank.

Mills AJ (1993). The cost of the district hospital: a case study in Malawi. *Bulletin of the World Health Organization,* 71(3–4):329–339.

Ojo K et al. (1995). *Cost analysis of health services in Sierra Leone. Annex III: A case study of Connaught Hospital and Waterloo Community Health Centre.* Geneva, World Health Organization (unpublished document; available on request from Department of Health in Sustainable Development, World Health Organization, 1211 Geneva 27, Switzerland).

Olave M, Montano Z (1993). *Unit cost and financial analysis for the Hospital 12 de abril, Bolivia.* Boston, MA, Management Sciences for Health (Health Financing and Sustainability Small Applied Research Report, No. 11).

Puglisi R, Bicknell WJ (1990). *Functional expenditure analysis: final report for Queen Elizabeth II Hospital, Maseru, Lesotho.* Boston, MA, Health Policy Institute, Boston University. [Includes two diskettes with their step-down analysis: one can be adapted by reader, one is write-protected.]

RAND Corporation (1992). *Unit cost analysis: a manual for facility administrators and policy-makers (Working draft).* Santa Monica, CA, RAND Corporation (Document WD-6282-MOH/RI).

Raymond S et al. (1987). *Financing and costs of health services in Belize.* Setauket, NY, International Resources Group Ltd.

Robertson R, Barona B, Pabon R (1977). Hospital cost accounting and analysis: the case of Candelaria. *Journal of community health,* 3(1):61–79.

Russell S, Gwynne G, Trisolini M (1988). *Health care financing in St. Lucia and costs of Victoria Hospital.* Stony Brook, NY, State University of New York at Stony Brook.

Salah H (1995). *Cost analysis for hospital care: summary output of Alexandria, Suez and Bani Suef General Hospitals. Preliminary results 1993–94.* Boston, MA, Harvard University School of Public Health.

Shepard DS (1988). *Analysis and recommendations on health financing in Rwanda.* Cambridge, MA, Harvard Institute for International Development.

Telyukov A (1995). *A guide to methodology: integrated system of cost accounting and analysis for inpatient care providers, developed and implemented at the Tomsk Oblast Teaching Hospital.* Bethesda, MD, Abt Associates Inc.

Trisolini MG et al. (1992). Methods for cost analysis, cost recovery and cost control for a public hospital in a developing country: Victoria Hospital, St. Lucia. *International journal of health planning and management,* 7:103–132.

Weaver M, Wong H, Sako AS et al. (1994). Prospects for reform of hospital fees in sub-Saharan Africa: a case study of Niamey National Hospital in Niger. *Social science and medicine,* 38(4):565–574.

Wong H (1989). *Cost analysis of Niamey Hospital.* Bethesda, MD, Abt Associates. [Niger].

Wong H (1993). *Health financing in Tuvalu.* Bethesda, MD, Abt Associates (Health Financing and Sustainability Project Technical Report, No. 11).

Zaman S (1993). *Cost analysis for hospital care: the case of Embaba Hospital, Cairo, Egypt.* Bethesda, MD, Abt Associates (Health Financing and Sustainability Project Technical Note, No. 32).

Other studies

Buve A, Foster S (1995). Carrying out a bed census at a district hospital in Zambia. *Heath policy and planning,* 10(4):441–445.

Institute for Health Policy Studies (1996). *The proper function of teaching hospitals within health systems.* Geneva, World Health Organization (unpublished document WHO/SHS/DHS/96.1; available on request from Department of Health Systems, World Health Organization, 1211 Geneva 27, Switzerland) and Paris, Flammarion Médecine-Sciences (French version).

Koné T et al. (1996). Expenditures on AIDS in Côte d'Ivoire. In: Ainsworth M, Over AM, Franzen L, eds. *Confronting AIDS: evidence from the developing world.* Brussels, European Commission AIDS Programme.

Jamison DT et al., eds. (1993). *Disease control priorities in developing countries.* New York, Oxford University Press for the World Bank.

Ma C-T, McGuire A, McGuire TG (1993). Paying for joint costs in health care. *Journal of economics and management strategy,* 2(1):71–95.

Mann J, Tarantola D, eds. (1996). *AIDS in the World II.* New York, Oxford University Press.

Shepard DS (1996). Expenditures on HIV/AIDS: levels and determinants — lessons from five countries. In: Ainsworth M, Over AM, Franzen L, eds. *Confronting AIDS: evidence from the developing world.* Brussels, European Commission AIDS Programme.

Shepard DS, Gonzales MC (1982). *A procedure for projecting hospital recurrent costs.* Boston, MA, Harvard School of Public Health, Department of Health Policy and Management (mimeograph).

Shepard DS et al. (1993). Cost–effectiveness of ambulatory surgery in Cali, Colombia. *Health policy and planning*, 8(2):136–142.

Shepard DS, Halstead SB (1993). Dengue (with notes on yellow fever and Japanese encephalitis). In: Jamison DT et al., eds. *Disease control priorities for developing countries*. New York, Oxford University Press for the World Bank, pp. 303–320.

Stansfield S, Shepard DS (1993). Acute respiratory infection. In: Jamison DT et al., eds. *Disease control priorities for developing countries*. New York, Oxford University Press for the World Bank, pp. 67–90.

Stryckman B (1996). *A comparative analysis of cost, resource use and financing of district health services in sub-Saharan Africa and Asia*. New York, UNICEF (Bamako Initiative Technical Report Series, No. 37).

Van Lerberghe W, Lafort Y (1990). The role of the hospital in the district: delivering or supporting primary health care? *Current Concerns, SHS Paper No. 2*. Geneva, World Health Organization (unpublished document WHO/SHS/CC/90.2; available on request from Department of Health Systems, World Health Organization, 1211 Geneva 27, Switzerland).

World Health Organization (1987). *Hospitals and health for all. Report of a WHO Expert Committee on the Role of Hospitals at the First Referral Level*. Geneva, World Health Organization (WHO Technical Report Series, No.744).

World Health Organization (1992). *The hospital in rural and urban districts. Report of a WHO Study Group on the Functions of Hospitals at the First Referral Level*. Geneva, World Health Organization (WHO Technical Report Series, No. 819).

Appendix 1

Tables for computing unit cost at Hospital X

Table A1. Costs by line item and source of
payment

Line item	Payment source			
	Ministry of Health	**Donor**	**Drug agency**	**Total cost**
Salary Director	10000			10000
Secretary	5000			5000
Handyman	1000			1000
Cleaner	1000			1000
Pharmacist	5000			5000
Physician 1	6000			6000
Physician 2	6000			6000
Physician 3		6000		6000
Nurse 1	5000			5000
Nurse 2	5000			5000
Nurse 3	5000			5000
Auxiliary	3000			3000
Drugs			20000	20000
Cleaning supplies	10000			10000
Other supplies	8000	4000		12000
Total	**70000**	**10000**	**20000**	**100000**

Table A2. Assignment of line item costs to cost centres

	Cost to be assigned	Cost centres						Total	%
		1. Overhead			2. Final				
		Administration	Cleaning	Pharmacy	Medicine	Surgery	Maternity		
Salary									
Director	10000	10000						10000	100
Secretary	5000	5000						5000	100
Handyman	1000	1000						1000	100
Cleaner	1000		1000					1000	100
Pharmacist	5000			5000				5000	100
Physician 1	6000				6000			6000	100
Physician 1	6000				1200	4800		6000	100
Physician 1	6000				1200		4800	6000	100
Nurse 1	5000				5000			5000	100
Nurse 2	5000					5000		5000	100
Nurse 3	5000						5000	5000	100
Auxiliary	3000				1200	1200	600	3000	100
Drugs	20000			12000	3200	2000	2800	20000	100
Cleaning supplies	10000		10000					10000	100
Other supplies	12000	12000						12000	100
Total	**100000**	**28000**	**11000**	**17000**	**17800**	**13000**	**13200**	**100000**	**100**

Table A3. Allocation of costs to final cost centres

Cost centre	Direct expense	Administration			Cleaning			Pharmacy		
		Allocation statistic Direct expense %	Expense reallocated	Revised direct expense	Allocation statistic Floor area %	Expense reallocated	Revised direct expense	Allocation statistic Pharmacy expense %	Expense reallocated	Revised direct expense
Overhead										
Admin.	28 000	100	28 000							
Cleaning	11 000	15	4 278	15 278	100	15 278				
Pharmacy	17 000	24	6 611	23 611	10	1 528	25 139	100	25 139	
Final										
Medicine	17 800	25	6 922	24 722	20	3 056	27 778	40	10 056	37 833
Surgery	13 000	18	5 056	18 056	30	4 583	22 639	25	6 285	28 924
Maternity	13 200	18	5 133	18 333	40	6 111	24 444	35	8 799	33 243
Total	**100 000**			**100 000**			**100 000**			**100 000**

Table A4. Unit cost calculation (pharmacy costs allocated)

	Inpatient days	Direct cost	Total cost	Cost per day		Ratio of total fully/partially	Direct as % of total
				Direct	Total		
Medicine	500	17800	37833	35.60	75.67	1.36	47
Surgery	300	13000	28924	43.33	96.41	1.28	45
Maternity	450	13200	33243	29.33	73.87	1.36	40
Total	**1250**	**44000**	**100000**	**35.20**	**80.00**	**1.34**	**44**

Table A5. Unit cost calculation (pharmacy costs *not* allocated)

	Units	Direct cost	Total cost	Cost per unit		Ratio of fully/partially	Direct as % of total
				Direct	Total		
Pharmacy	5000	17000	25139	3.40	5.03		68
Medicine	500	17800	27778	35.60	55.56	1.36	64
Surgery	300	13000	22639	43.33	75.46	1.28	57
Maternity	450	13200	24444	29.33	54.32	1.36	54
Subtotal	**1250**	**44000**	**74861**	**35.20**	**59.89**	**1.34**	**59**

Appendix 2

Step-down allocation using direct cost

An approximate cost analysis can be carried out by allocating indirect costs on the basis of each department's percentage share of direct costs, though this is recommended only when other data are not available for allocating direct costs. This approach is commonly used for assigning costs of the hospital's administration, and occasionally for overhead costs (as in Kutzin's Jamaica study). The approach is substantially simpler than the detailed step-down described in Chapter 1, and does not require information about floor area, bed-days etc. One can therefore legitimately ask how inaccurate is an allocation based on direct costs only. Does it introduce systematic biases that can be offset by the use of adjustment factors? For example, if prior studies show that the direct-cost approach typically overstates unit cost of inpatient wards by 20%, one would know that one should deflate unit costs by that amount when using the method.

To compare the direct-cost method with more sophisticated approaches, data from previous step-down studies were reanalysed. Where possible, a revised unit cost was calculated using the direct-cost method. The results were then compared with those reported in each original study. Table A6 presents the comparison of the two methods, by study and by department. The comparison is expressed as a ratio of unit costs by method. For example, an entry of 1.4 indicates that unit costs appear 40% higher using the direct-cost method, compared with the method used by the study authors.

Table A7 summarizes results across the 12 studies that were reanalysed. The results confirm that the direct-cost method tends to understate unit costs for inpatient care (in 10 out of 12 studies) and to overstate costs for outpatient care (at least in studies where ancillary costs centres were allocated). The discrepancy occurs because inpatient wards use a lot of costly indirect resources such as kitchen and laundry, beyond the share one would predict on the basis of direct cost. Equivalently, outpatient services use a relatively low share of these resources. An exception to this pattern is the operating theatre, where the direct-cost method overstates unit costs (presumably because most of the theatre's costs were easy to assign before the step-down allocation, leaving it only a small share of indirect cost).

Table A6. Comparison across studies: unit cost using direct-cost method, as a proportion of unit cost reported in study[a,b]

	Papua New Guinea		Saint Lucia	Jamaica	Lesotho	Sierra Leone	Gambia		Egypt	Dominica	Montserrat	Bhutan (Thimphu)
	Hospital 1	Hospital 2					Hospital 1	Hospital 2				
ALL INPATIENT	0.994	0.928	0.905	1.013	0.958	0.241	0.93	1.072	0.812	0.936	0.951	0.956
Medicine/surgery					0.902					0.829	0.877	
Medicine	1.279	0.927	0.896	1.113		0.234	1.088	1.213	0.848			
ICU[c]	1.464					0.785			0.327			
Medicine, not ICU	1.189					0.188			1.353	0.911		0.768
Surgery	0.510	0.645					0.796	1.202	0.621			
Excluding theatre			0.906	0.964		0.259				0.753		0.781
Theatre only			1.180		1.665	1.621					1.042	1.217
Obstetrics/gynaecology	0.994	1.039	0.932	0.807	0.999		0.800	0.909	0.730	1.026	1.017	0.904
Obstetrics only	0.930	1.062	0.939									
Gynaecology only	1.276	0.977	0.920									
Paediatrics	1.124	1.002	0.843	1.116	0.647	0.179	0.836	0.927	1.296	0.927	0.977	0.883
Private			0.888									
Outpatient	0.756	1.083	1.067	0.957	0.769	1.451			1.424	0.989	0.919	0.918
Outpatient casualty					0.807		1.171					
Outpatient clinics					0.619			0.588				
Drugs allocated?	y		y	y	y	n	y	y	y	n	n	y
X-ray, lab. allocated?	y		n	y	y	n	y	y	y	n	n	n

Notes: [a] Direct-cost method uses each final cost centre's share of the direct cost as the basis for allocating indirect cost.
[b] Original methods used other bases for allocation. In some cases, categories in the original study were combined to make results comparable.
[c] Intensive care unit.

Table A7. Summary across studies: unit cost using direct-cost method, as a proportion of unit cost reported in study

Service	Observations	Number of observations where using direct-cost method makes unit cost lower or higher		Mean value	Standard deviation
		Lower	Higher		
ALL INPATIENT	12	10	2	0.891	0.205
Medicine/surgery	3	3	0	0.869	0.030
Medicine	8	4	4	0.950	0.306
Medicine, not ICU[a]	5	3	2	0.882	0.403
ICU	3	2	1	0.859	0.467
Surgery	5	4	1	0.755	0.241
Excluding theatre	5	5	0	0.733	0.249
Theatre only	5	0	5	1.345	0.251
Obstetrics/gynaecology	9	6	3	0.928	0.100
Obstetrics only	5	4	1	0.947	0.085
Gynaecology only	3	2	1	1.058	0.156
Paediatrics	12	8	4	0.896	0.268
Private	1	1	0	0.888	0.000
Outpatient	10	6	4	1.033	0.226
Outpatient casualty	1	1	0	0.807	0.000
Outpatient clinics	3	2	1	0.793	0.268

[a] Intensive care unit.

The results across studies differ substantially, however, especially at the level of individual wards. It is not clear what would be a reasonable adjustment factor for paediatrics; the direct-cost method can lead one to a unit cost which is 30% too high or 36% too low, depending on the study. This variation may come about because the studies differed in many respects that could not be controlled for, including the specific step-down approach that they used originally and the type of costs allocated. As a method for allocating costs, the direct-cost approach should probably be a last resort to be used only when other data are not available for allocating indirect costs. On the other hand, it is useful to compute allocation using both methods and to compare the results. If, for instance, one ward has much higher costs using the direct-cost approach than using the step-down approach, investigating the reason for this may help one to understand the sources of cost differences between wards (e.g. which wards use a lot of kitchen or laundry services).

Appendix 3

Table of annualization factors

Table A8. Annualization factors

Useful life (years)											Discount rate										
	0%	1%	2%	3%	4%	5%	6%	7%	8%	9%	10%	11%	12%	13%	14%	15%	16%	17%	18%	19%	20%
1		0.990	0.980	0.971	0.962	0.952	0.943	0.935	0.926	0.917	0.909	0.901	0.893	0.885	0.877	0.870	0.862	0.855	0.847	0.840	0.833
2		1.970	1.942	1.913	1.886	1.859	1.833	1.808	1.783	1.759	1.736	1.713	1.690	1.668	1.647	1.626	1.605	1.585	1.566	1.547	1.528
3		2.941	2.884	2.829	2.775	2.723	2.673	2.624	2.577	2.531	2.487	2.444	2.402	2.361	2.322	2.283	2.246	2.210	2.174	2.140	2.106
4		3.902	3.808	3.717	3.630	3.546	3.465	3.387	3.312	3.240	3.170	3.102	3.037	2.974	2.914	2.855	2.798	2.743	2.690	2.639	2.589
5		4.853	4.713	4.580	4.452	4.329	4.212	4.100	3.993	3.890	3.791	3.696	3.605	3.517	3.433	3.352	3.274	3.199	3.127	3.058	2.991
6		5.795	5.601	5.417	5.242	5.076	4.917	4.767	4.623	4.486	4.355	4.231	4.111	3.998	3.889	3.784	3.685	3.589	3.498	3.410	3.326
7		6.728	6.472	6.230	6.002	5.786	5.582	5.389	5.206	5.033	4.868	4.712	4.564	4.423	4.288	4.160	4.039	3.922	3.812	3.706	3.605
8		7.652	7.325	7.020	6.733	6.463	6.210	5.971	5.747	5.535	5.335	5.146	4.968	4.799	4.639	4.487	4.344	4.207	4.078	3.954	3.837
9		8.566	8.162	7.786	7.435	7.108	6.802	6.515	6.247	5.995	5.759	5.537	5.328	5.132	4.946	4.772	4.607	4.451	4.303	4.163	4.031
10		9.471	8.983	8.530	8.111	7.722	7.360	7.024	6.710	6.418	6.145	5.889	5.650	5.426	5.216	5.019	4.833	4.659	4.494	4.339	4.192
11		10.368	9.787	9.253	8.760	8.306	7.887	7.499	7.139	6.805	6.495	6.207	5.938	5.687	5.453	5.234	5.029	4.836	4.656	4.486	4.327
12		11.255	10.575	9.954	9.385	8.863	8.384	7.943	7.536	7.161	6.814	6.492	6.194	5.918	5.660	5.421	5.197	4.988	4.793	4.611	4.439
13		12.134	11.348	10.635	9.986	9.394	8.853	8.358	7.904	7.487	7.103	6.750	6.424	6.122	5.842	5.583	5.342	5.118	4.910	4.715	4.533
14		13.004	12.106	11.296	10.563	9.899	9.295	8.745	8.244	7.786	7.367	6.982	6.628	6.302	6.002	5.724	5.468	5.229	5.008	4.802	4.611
15		13.865	12.849	11.938	11.118	10.380	9.712	9.108	8.559	8.061	7.606	7.191	6.811	6.462	6.142	5.847	5.575	5.324	5.092	4.876	4.675
16		14.718	13.578	12.561	11.652	10.838	10.106	9.447	8.851	8.313	7.824	7.379	6.974	6.604	6.265	5.954	5.668	5.405	5.162	4.938	4.730
17		15.562	14.292	13.166	12.166	11.274	10.477	9.763	9.122	8.544	8.022	7.549	7.120	6.729	6.373	6.047	5.749	5.475	5.222	4.990	4.775
18		16.398	14.992	13.754	12.659	11.690	10.828	10.059	9.372	8.756	8.201	7.702	7.250	6.840	6.467	6.128	5.818	5.534	5.273	5.033	4.812
19		17.226	15.678	14.324	13.134	12.085	11.158	10.336	9.604	8.950	8.365	7.839	7.366	6.938	6.550	6.198	5.877	5.584	5.316	5.070	4.843
20		18.046	16.351	14.877	13.590	12.462	11.470	10.594	9.818	9.129	8.514	7.963	7.469	7.025	6.623	6.259	5.929	5.628	5.353	5.101	4.870
21		18.857	17.011	15.415	14.029	12.821	11.764	10.836	10.017	9.292	8.649	8.075	7.562	7.102	6.687	6.312	5.973	5.665	5.384	5.127	4.891
22		19.660	17.658	15.937	14.451	13.163	12.042	11.061	10.201	9.442	8.772	8.176	7.645	7.170	6.743	6.359	6.011	5.696	5.410	5.149	4.909
23		20.456	18.292	16.444	14.857	13.489	12.303	11.272	10.371	9.580	8.883	8.266	7.718	7.230	6.792	6.399	6.044	5.723	5.432	5.167	4.925
24		21.243	18.914	16.936	15.247	13.799	12.550	11.469	10.529	9.707	8.985	8.348	7.784	7.283	6.835	6.434	6.073	5.746	5.451	5.182	4.937
25		22.023	19.523	17.413	15.622	14.094	12.783	11.654	10.675	9.823	9.077	8.422	7.843	7.330	6.873	6.464	6.097	5.766	5.467	5.195	4.948
26		22.795	20.121	17.877	15.983	14.375	13.003	11.826	10.810	9.929	9.161	8.488	7.896	7.372	6.906	6.491	6.118	5.783	5.480	5.206	4.956
27		23.560	20.707	18.327	16.330	14.643	13.211	11.987	10.935	10.027	9.237	8.548	7.943	7.409	6.935	6.514	6.136	5.798	5.492	5.215	4.964
28		24.316	21.281	18.764	16.663	14.898	13.406	12.137	11.051	10.116	9.307	8.602	7.984	7.441	6.961	6.534	6.152	5.810	5.502	5.223	4.970
29		25.066	21.844	19.188	16.984	15.141	13.591	12.278	11.158	10.198	9.370	8.650	8.022	7.470	6.983	6.551	6.166	5.820	5.510	5.229	4.975
30		25.808	22.396	19.600	17.292	15.372	13.765	12.409	11.258	10.274	9.427	8.694	8.055	7.496	7.003	6.566	6.177	5.829	5.517	5.235	4.979

Appendix 4

Exercises[1]

Exercise 1. A district hospital in Bangladesh

Note: This exercise applies the principles of cost analysis and income analysis at the level of an individual hospital, providing the reader with an opportunity to calculate unit costs and practise other skills from Chapters 1 and 2.

A typical district hospital in Bangladesh has 50 beds and 74 staff (14 physicians, 26 nurses, 15 technicians and skilled staff, and 19 unskilled support staff). This type of hospital has three patient care cost centres — inpatient wards, theatre (for surgical operations), and outpatient department (for both clinics and casualty services). Four intermediate cost centres were used — ambulance, X-ray, pharmacy, and laboratory. Because of the simplicity of the hospital, only one overhead cost centre — administration — was defined; this subsumes other support functions such as security, cleaning, and maintenance.

Table A9 shows the annual direct costs of this hospital by cost centre. The average annual 1996 salary for each staff position plus benefits (rather than the individual salaries at a specific hospital) were used to estimate personnel costs. The exchange rate was 40 taka (Tk) to one US dollar. The average annual costs (including benefits amounting to 60% of base salaries) per staff are: Tk 89 000 (US\$ 2225) per physician, Tk 46 000 (US\$ 1150) per nurse, Tk 44 000

[1] The authors gratefully acknowledge assistance from Professor James Killingsworth, Mr Kawnine and Ms Tahmina Begum of the Bangladesh Health Economics Unit, and feedback from facilitators and participants in the workshops on hospital costing in Dhaka, Bangladesh, 26–28 May 1997. They also benefited from feedback from Thomas Zigora, Freckson Ropi and Ashley Ghisewe of Zimbabwe's Ministry of Health and Child Welfare and the other participants at a workshop on hospital costing in Harare, Zimbabwe, 23–24 October 1997. Additional exercises included here were developed for an international workshop on hospital costing held in Cairo, Egypt, 1–4 February 1999, for which the assistance of Dr Belgacem Sabri of the WHO Regional Office for the Eastern Mediterranean and Dr Hassan Salah of the Partnerships for Health Reform project is greatly appreciated. The authors are also grateful for the financial support of the United Kingdom's Department for International Development, and the support of the WHO representatives in Bangladesh, Egypt and Zimbabwe and of WHO in Geneva, Switzerland, and Alexandria, Egypt, in the development and testing of these exercises.

(US$ 1100) per technician or administrative staff member, Tk 23000 (US$ 575) per unskilled support staff member, and Tk 48000 (US$ 1200) per staff member overall. Personnel costs were attributed to each cost centre based on how the staff members spent their time. Non-personnel costs and capital costs incurred in a patient care or intermediate cost centre were assigned to that cost centre, while all other costs (general maintenance and the annualized capital cost of the buildings and furnishings) were assigned to administration. Ambulance operations and "other" expenses, including utilities (for which fuel and equipment are imported), account for high shares of expenses because of the extent to which they rely on imports.

Exercise 1a

Calculate the total cost of each cost centre (treating all the intermediate and patient care cost centres as final cost centres) by completing the blank cells in Table A9.

Table A9. Allocating overhead costs to cost centres

Cost centre	Direct expense[a] US$	Allocation statistic	Allocation %	Allocated expense US$	Total expense US$
Overhead:					
Administration and other	34902	direct cost	0.0	0	0
Intermediate:					
Ambulance, etc.	12804				
X-ray	6199				
Pharmacy	11737				
Laboratory	9134				
Patient care:					
Inpatient wards	30582				
Theatre	14811				
Outpatient department	11054				
Total	131223				

[a] Converted at the 1997 official exchange rate of 40 Bangladeshi taka to one US dollar.

Exercise 1b

Calculate the unit cost of each final cost centre, a target fee for a typical unit of service by that cost centre, and the potential revenue generated by that cost centre by completing the blank cells in Table A10.

Hint: The target fee percentage is the proportion of the average unit cost which is charged to paying patients, and the target fee is the unit cost multiplied by the target fee percentage. The percentage of patients charged is the share of patients not exempted from payment. The collection efficiency is the share of fees imposed that are actually collected from patients and officially remitted to the hospital. The total revenue from each cost centre is the cost (the product of the volume of service multiplied by its unit cost) multiplied by the three factors discussed on pages 43–44. The hospital administration sets the fee in each cost centre equal to the target fee percentage of the unit cost. However, not all patients are actually charged the set fee. Some are exempted due to poverty or other considerations.

Exercise 1c

The hospital needs to recover one-quarter of its total costs from user fees. Determine whether the assumptions above will enable it to meet this target. If it will not, suggest an alternative set of values that will.

Hint: Add the revenues from each final cost centre in Table A10 and compare the sum to the total costs of the hospital. Raising any of the percentages will raise the total; lowering any will lower the total. The impact will be greater if the percentages are changed on the larger sources of revenue.

Table A10. Calculating unit costs and potential cost recovery

Final cost centre	Total expense (US$)	Volume	Units	Unit cost (US$)	Target fee %	Target fee (US$)	Patients charged %	Collection efficiency %	Potential revenue (US$)
Intermediate:									
Ambulance	17 444	20 000	kilometers		60		90	80	
X-ray	8 445	4 000	films		60		80	90	
Pharmacy	15 990	30 000	scripts		75		60	90	
Laboratory	12 444	50 000	tests		50		80	90	
Patient care:									
Inpatient wards	41 663	15 000	days		30		70	70	
Theatre	20 178	2 000	operations		20		80	80	
Outpatient department	15 059	20 000	visits		60		70	80	
Total	131 223								

Exercise 2. Should we contract out laundry services?

Note: This case compares internal hospital laundry services (with either owned or leased equipment) with outsourced laundry services.

As a hospital administrator, you are constantly challenged to deliver quality services efficiently. This objective includes deciding when to make capital expenditure (i.e. expenditure that is expected to provide benefits for longer than one year). Such a decision now has to be made regarding the laundry department.

Your major piece of equipment in this department has become more and more unreliable. It now breaks down so often that you never know when it will be working. Linen is often not as clean as it should be and the state of employees' uniforms is embarrassing. Working conditions in the laundry are deplorable, and current space is too small to house the equipment — new or old. Laundry employees are disgruntled because of these conditions; they take great pride in their work. You know that some hospitals in the region have contracted out their laundry services. Some hospitals have been pleased with the results while others doubt the long-term benefits.

The current equipment is completely depreciated and outmoded. The capital cost of refurbishing the laundry would be as follows:

	US$
Renovation of laundry building	30 000
New equipment	65 000
Total capital cost	95 000

The expected life of the equipment and the renovation is assumed to be 20 years. The inflation rate is 7%, the real interest rate is 3%, and the nominal interest rate is about 10%. In addition, a rural hospital in the next town is willing to buy your outmoded equipment for US$ 2000 to use as a back-up to its own washing machine.

Currently, the variable cost (for soap, water, utilities and direct labour) is US$ 0.03 per kg, and your hospital processes 300 000 kg of laundry per year. Your annual fixed operating costs are:

	US$
Maintenance	1400
Administrative salaries	8000
Total fixed costs	9400

A company with three years' experience has indicated that it would be prepared to collect the laundry, wash it at its own facility and return it to the hospital for US$ 0.06 per kg (rising annually with inflation) if it were to get the contract to do so. In-house administrative oversight of a contract would cost the hospital US$ 2000. Alternatively, the company is willing to refurbish the space and lease the equipment to the hospital at US$ 10 000 per year — renewable annually for up to 20 years with the annual lease payment rising at the rate of inflation. The hospital would be responsible for all variable costs and maintenance.

Exercise 2

a. *Given this information, identify the three options contained in the description above.*

b. *For each option, estimate the capital costs, operating (both fixed and variable) costs, and total costs.*

c. *Choose the best option in terms of the lowest annualized costs.*

d. Discuss other features of the best option (e.g. flexibility, future cost expectations, reliability).

e. Identify at least one more option, not mentioned above, which could also be considered.

Exercise 3. A missed opportunity

Note: This case deals with preparation of a cost analysis at the level of a hospital, identifying all the departments affected, and interpreting the results for hospital policy.

As the administrator of a crowded but respected provincial public hospital, you have calculated that, by the end of this fiscal year, your hospital should be operating at a surplus. If you make no changes, your hospital's costs will be US$ 15 000 less than its budget from the national government and you will need to return this balance to the government. As an experienced administrator, you know that if you return the funds you will miss an opportunity to improve services.

Dr Vivek, chief surgeon at your hospital, has just heard the good news. He approaches you before you can draft the memo to other department heads informing them of this opportunity and requesting their immediate input. With a tone of urgency, Dr Vivek asks that the hospital should purchase new endoscopy equipment that detects and replaces the surgical treatment of colon cancer. The equipment is estimated to cost US$ 10 000. Dr Vivek tells you that this cost is "minimal" and he sees no reason why his request should not be approved for funding.

After discussing this matter with Dr Vivek for two hours and after talking to a friend who is a financial analyst at a nearby hospital, you realize that there are other costs involved in purchasing this new piece of equipment. Dr Vivek could give only "soft numbers" when you asked him how many patients with colon cancer were treated on an inpatient and outpatient basis in the hospital in each of the last three years and, of those, how many could have benefited from the proposed equipment. According to Dr Vivek, around 500 patients a year could benefit from the new equipment — about half are patients now receiving other diagnostic procedures only and half are patients receiving both diagnostic procedures and surgical treatment. Without the new equipment, each of the surgical cases would spend a week in the hospital. If they do not need to be admitted, their place would be taken by other elective surgical patients who usually wait several weeks for admission.

With your friend's help and Dr Vivek's information, you estimate the full capital costs as follows:

	US$
New endoscopy equipment (10-year life)	10 000
Expanded outpatient treatment room (20-year life)	5000
Total capital costs	15 000

Your friend advises you that the necessary approvals to apply the US$ 15 000 anticipated surplus to these capital costs could be obtained if you make an adequate case.

The inflation rate is 7% and the real interest rate is 3% per year. Variable costs are: physician (0.25 of annual salary of US$ 10 000), technician (0.5 of annual salary of US$ 3000), nurse (0.5 of annual salary of US$ 5000), and supplies (US$ 4500 per year). Your analysis is based on the principle of fully allocated costs. That is, it is assumed that staff and facilities are being utilized as intensively as they can be, given existing salaries, working conditions and supervision. While it may theoretically be possible for existing hospital staff to perform more services, in practice managerial changes and incentives that are beyond the scope of the proposed new service would be needed to achieve such gains. Fixed annual operating costs are maintenance (US$ 500) and salaries (US$ 1000).

Dr Vivek foresees a charge of US$ 25 for patients receiving diagnosis only, and US$ 50 per patient receiving diagnosis and treatment. Because of free care and incomplete collection of fees, net revenue will be half of these amounts.

Exercise 3

a. Determine the annualized costs of Dr Vivek's proposal, counting all fixed and variable costs, and compare them to his original US$ 10 000 estimate.
b. Discuss how this project might affect costs in other patient care units.
c. Estimate the net income from the new procedure. Compare net income and costs and indicate the impact on the hospital's finances.
d. Discuss whether benefits to the health of the hospital's patients justify these costs.
e. If the capital costs of the new service are financed through the surplus, would the annualized costs be zero?

Exercise 4. The wish list

Note: This case deals with thinking quantitatively about the costs of a new service, and qualitatively about its contribution to the facility's goals.

The Ministry of Health has asked each hospital to submit details of one capital improvement project that its administration wishes to be funded. Improvement projects can range from beautifying one or all wards to adding a new medical service or opening a new operating theatre. No dollar limit has been given, but the instructions state that you are to submit a financial feasibility statement showing all projected costs and revenues within a three-year time frame, and that you should not exceed an allowable net increase in operating cost of 1% of the hospital's operating budget, including annualized capital costs. It is noted that the funds from the ministry are "one-time only", implying that costs beyond the 1% guideline will need to be self-financed.

Exercise 4

Think of a capital improvement project for your hospital. Describe the types of data you would obtain to determine whether the impact is worth the cost of achieving it.

Exercise 5. Data sources and analysis

As the financial analyst in the Ministry of Health, you have been asked to check on Baba Hospital's estimated drug costs per admission for the recently completed fiscal year. Officials at the Ministry of Health feel that the hospital administrator's own estimates are inaccurate, both in terms of the overall average drug cost per admission and in the breakdown by each of the three wards (medicine, surgical, maternity). For the purpose of this exercise, assume that outpatients do not receive drugs and can be ignored.

One problem with the administrator's estimates is that they are based only on records of drugs purchased through official requisitions to the state pharmaceutical purchasing board. In reality, hospital staff often buy drugs locally (or on the private market) when emergencies arise, or when the state board runs out of certain drugs. The administrator did not know the amount of "unofficial" drugs purchased and counted only the US$ 900 000 in officially purchased drugs. The head pharmacist maintains a separate log that includes invoices on all drug purchases (i.e. official and unofficial) but the hospital administrator forgot this.

Your first task is to estimate the expenditures on "unofficial" drug purchases during the year. Your data source is a 60 cm-deep file drawer in the hospital pharmacy, which is full of paper invoices for all drugs obtained over the year. It would be extremely time-consuming to enter all these invoices into a database, so you decide to sample.

> a. *What two pieces of information do you need to obtain from the sample?*
> b. *Suggest a sampling approach to estimate these two pieces of information.*

Suppose you use a ruler to divide the invoices into 20 equal batches of 3 cm each, which you then mark with a paperclip. Then, in order to estimate the total number of invoices for the year, suppose you arbitrarily choose two of the batches and count the number of invoices in each batch (which turn out to be 98 and 102). You also randomly choose a percentage between 0 and 100 — e.g. 37%. By putting a mark on your ruler at 1.11 cm (37% of the 3 cm width of each batch), you quickly sample the invoice that is 37% of the way down each batch. Suppose the sampling results tell you that the average amount per invoice is:

	US$
Official drugs	440
Unofficial drugs	105
Total	545

c. *Using the total number of invoices per year, what is the amount of "unofficial drug purchases"? Is the estimate of US$ 900 000 for official drugs plausible? What is your estimate of the total being spent on both official and unofficial drugs, and what percentage is being spent on each?*

d. *Assuming that there were 12 000 hospital admissions in the most recent fiscal year, what is the average drug cost per admission?*

e. *Assuming that the proportional breakdown of drug cost per clinical department for each of the three wards (medicine, surgical, maternity) is 33%, 50% and 17% respectively, what is the total cost for each of these clinical services? What is the average drug cost per admission for each clinical service?*

Assume that you do not know the proportional breakdown of total drug costs across the three inpatient departments. Another problem presented to you as the Ministry of Health's financial analyst is that the hospital administrator did not have computerized data showing which wards were responsible for each drug purchase. She therefore estimated drug costs for each ward by allocating the total drug cost in proportion to each ward's share of the total inpatient floor space. As a result, she predicts the following drug costs per admission:

Administrator's estimate of official drug costs per admission, by ward

Ward	Floor space of each ward (m²)	Distribution of floor space (%)	Estimated total drug cost (US$)	Admissions	Drug cost per admission (US$)
Medicine	250	25	225 000	3 000	75.00
Surgery	360	36	324 000	4 000	81.00
Maternity	390	39	351 000	5 000	70.20
Overall	1000	100	900 000	12 000	75.00

f. *Do you think floor space is a reliable measure of drug use? If not, what do you think is an appropriate measure?*

You doubt that the maternity ward could really have incurred higher drug costs than the surgical ward. You think you can improve on the hospital's estimates. Your data source is a box full of requisition forms submitted to the hospital pharmacy by the wards, filed in approximate chronological order. Each requisition shows the name of the drug, the quantity, and the ward that placed the request. Again, the box is large, so you decide to sample the requisitions randomly and pull out 20 records. You summarize the information in the following table (for simplicity, we assume there are only three drugs):

Number of bottles distributed by ward

	Drug A	Drug B	Drug C
Quantity for:			
Medicine	100	50	40
Surgery	80	30	20
Maternity	70	50	10

The requisitions do not show price, so you assume that each drug costs the amount usually charged by the state purchasing board. The prices per bottle are therefore $ 5 for drug A, $ 10 for drug B and $ 20 for drug C.

g. *Combine the prices and quantities to compute the total value of drugs purchased by each ward for the 20 sampled records.*

h. *Compute each ward's share of drug costs for this sample. Apply these shares to the total drug cost you computed earlier in order to estimate the total drug cost by ward.*

i. *Divide each ward's drug costs by its admission volume to obtain the drug cost per admission by ward. How do these numbers compare with the hospital's own estimates? Does it seem reasonable to allocate drug costs on the basis of each ward's share of floor space as the hospital administrator did?*

Exercise 6. Hospital reform case study

The state of Caribana is on the brink of health reform. Its Ministry of Health is currently designing a system of national health insurance expected to cover almost all of the country's residents. Persons insured under this system are to be covered for "essential hospital services". A new national health insurance organization will collect premiums from individuals and employers (and from government on behalf of the poor) and will pay hospitals. Essential hospital services, while not yet defined in detail, are expected to include a limited set of common and cost-effective treatments, such as deliveries (both ordinary and complicated), treatment of respiratory infections, appendectomy and other emergency surgery, and so on. General government revenues will continue to fund primary care services in public facilities and will also be used to cover highly specialized and expensive tertiary care in the country's major referral hospitals. Private physicians' services will continue to be paid for by voluntary private insurance or by patients themselves.

Currently, almost all of the country's hospitals are run by the Ministry of Health or by a regional health authority. Almost all (95%) of their funding comes from those sources, and only 5% comes from so-called "cost recovery" (private insurance and patient fees). While the ministry and health authorities would like to increase revenue from cost recovery, they have so far succeeded only with outpatient services and drugs. With regard to inpatient services, they fear that if fees approach the real economic costs and exemptions become difficult to obtain, the services may become prohibitively expensive. If that happened, ordinary citizens would not be able to afford hospital care (or would experience financial hardship if they paid for it). Under a system of health insurance, hospitals could raise their inpatient fees and reduce their dependence on government subsidy while preserving access to needed hospital care.

Your assignment is to advise the government, as it moves from concepts to specific plans, by answering the following questions:

a. *On what basis would you define essential hospital services (i.e. the benefit package of the proposed insurance plan), and what kind of system of hospital costing would be needed to support this?*

b. *How should the health insurance authority pay hospitals for services that are covered?*

c. *Based on your answers to the preceding questions, what are the implications for the level and rate of change of hospital costs?*

Answers

Answers to Exercise 1

1a. As overhead costs represent only about one-quarter of the hospital's total cost and comprise a range of overhead services, administrators felt that overhead costs could be assigned in proportion to the direct costs of the final (intermediate and patient care) cost centres. Thus, the direct cost of each final cost centre should be used as the allocation statistic. The allocation percentages should be calculated as the share of each cost centre in total direct expenses (less overhead direct expenses). The total costs of each final cost centre are the sum of its direct and allocated costs. The total costs should equal (except for possible rounding error) the sum of the overhead costs plus the direct costs of each cost centre.

Table A11 contains the answer to Exercise 1a.

Table A11. Allocating overhead costs to cost centres (US$)

Cost centre	Direct expense (US$)	Allocation statistic: direct cost	Allocation %	Allocated expense (US$)	Total expense (US$)
Overhead:					
Administrative and other	34 902	—	0.00	0	0
Intermediate:					
Ambulance, etc.	12 804	12 804	13.29	4 640	17 444
X-ray	6 199	6 199	6.44	2 246	8 445
Pharmacy	11 737	11 737	12.19	4 253	15 990
Laboratory	9 134	9 134	9.48	3 310	12 444
Patient care:					
Inpatient wards	30 582	30 582	31.75	11 081	41 663
Theatre	14 811	14 811	15.38	5 367	20 178
Outpatient department	11 054	11 054	11.48	4 005	15 059
Total	**131 223**	**96 321**	**100.00**	**34 902**	**131 223**

1b, 1c. Table A12 shows the answers to Exercises 1b and 1c.

Table A12. Calculating unit costs and potential cost recovery

Final cost centre	Total expense (US$)	Volume	Units	Unit cost (US$)	Target fee (%)	Target fee (US$)	Patients charged (%)	Collection efficiency (%)	Potential revenue (US$)
Intermediate:									
Ambulance	17 444	20 000	kilometers	0.87	60	0.52	90	80	7 536
X-ray	8 445	4 000	films	2.11	60	1.27	80	90	3 648
Pharmacy	15 990	30 000	scripts	0.53	75	0.40	60	90	6 476
Laboratory	12 444	50 000	tests	0.25	50	0.12	80	90	4 480
Patient care:									
Inpatient wards	41 663	15 000	days	2.78	30	0.83	70	70	6 124
Theatre	20 178	2 000	operations	10.09	20	2.02	80	80	2 583
Outpatient dept.	15 059	20 000	visits	0.75	60	0.45	70	80	5 060
Total	**131 223**								**35 907**

Based on these calculations, the hospital will recover 27% (35 907/ 131 223) of its costs through fees, slightly exceeding its target. While it may be possible to increase the amounts by increasing the target fee percentage, such increases may cause reductions in the percentage of patients from whom fees are actually collected (as higher fees may cause more exemptions). Alternatively, raising fee levels may simply lead to a reduction in the total number of patients, thereby reducing the effect of the fee increase on total revenues.

Answers to Exercise 2

2a. Failure to make the needed investment would mean discontinuing the service. Care should be exercised in identifying the choices. In this case, the three options for the hospital administrator are to maintain the laundry department as an in-house service with purchased new equipment, to contract an outside company to perform this service, or to lease the equipment from an outside company.

2b. First, we note that all three options involve a one-time income inflow of US$ 2000 from the sale of the old laundry equipment. We then examine the costs of each of these options in the order above. We present below the first-year costs, recognizing that they will rise by the rate of inflation.

- The capital cost of renovating and equipping the hospital's laundry facility is estimated to be US$ 95 000. We annualize this amount using the procedures in Box 1. Using 3% as the real interest rate, the annualization factor is 14.877. With an inflation rate of 7%, the replacement capital cost of the project at the end of the first year would be US$ 101 650 (US$ 95 000 × 1.07). The annualized capital cost is US$ 6833 (US$ 101 650 ÷ 14.877). Using the information above, total variable and fixed costs are:

	US$
Variable costs (0.03/kg × 300 000 kg)	9000
Fixed costs/year	
Annualized capital cost	6833
Maintenance and space costs	1400
Administrative salaries	8000
Total fixed and variable costs	25 233

The net first-year cost of the in-house option is US$ 23 233 (US$ 25 233 less the one-time income of US$ 2000 from selling the equipment). The second-year cost is US$ 26 999 (US$ 25 233 × 1.07). We assume that operating costs rise with inflation, and our method of annualizing the capital costs gives values that also rise with inflation.
- The next step in the analysis is to determine the cost of the second option, i.e. to contract a company to do the laundry services for the

hospital. Using the price quotation from a company of US$ 0.06 per kg, the cost of the second option is:

	US$
Contract fee (US$ 0.06 × 300 000 kg of laundry)	18 000
In-house administrative oversight of contract	2000
Total cost of contract	20 000

The net first-year cost of the contract option is US$ 18 000 (US$ 20 000 less the one-time income of US$ 2000 from selling the equipment). The second-year cost is US$ 21 400 (US$ 20 000 × 1.07), as the price in the renewable contract will rise with inflation.

- The leased equipment would entail:

	US$
Variable costs	9000
Fixed costs/year	
Lease payment	10 000
Maintenance and space costs	1400
Administrative salaries	8000
Total fixed and variable costs	28 400

The net first-year cost of the lease option is US$ 26 400 (US$ 28 400 less the one-time income of US$ 2000 from selling the equipment). The second-year cost is US$ 30 388 (US$ 28 400 × 1.07) as the lease fee and other costs will rise with inflation.

2c. The first-year costs of the three options can now be compared: US$ 23 233 (in-house option), US$ 18 000 (contract option) and US$ 26 400 (lease option). The second-year costs have the same relationship, without the one-time income inflow. The hospital administrator would then choose the least-cost option of contracting out the work (US$ 18 000). The lease option is most expensive in this example. The cost of each of these options, as we have calculated it, would rise at the annual rate of inflation (7% per year).

2d. The option of contracting out the work provides flexibility for the hospital if the laundry or the space it occupies needs change. A laundry service that is contracted out might achieve efficiencies through more productive staff, better management, economies of scale through larger equipment, better use of plant and equipment through multiple shifts, or lower labour costs. One liability of this approach is the risk that transport may be interrupted, whether by vehicle breakdown, bad weather, civil disturbance or war. If this risk of interruption is significant, the in-house option may be necessary (as it proved to be when this analysis was done in a hospital in wartime Beirut, Lebanon). Alternatively, additional inventory and storage could provide another way to ensure adequate laundry even if transportation is disrupted. Financing the in-house option might pose a significant challenge for the hospital. Although the hospital may have some capital reserves, public hospitals usually need special approval for this type of capital expenditure.

2e. Other options are to share laundry services with another hospital, or group of hospitals. The laundry could be based either at your hospital or at another. Or one could buy used equipment, or see whether limited renovation could keep the laundry functional for a few more years.

Answers to Exercise 3

3a. We first derive the annualized capital costs. Assuming a life of 10 years, the annualization factor for the new endoscopy equipment is 8.530. The annualized capital cost for the endoscopy equipment in the first year is US$ 1254 (calculated as US$ 10 000 × 1.07 = US$ 10 700; US$ 10 700 ÷ 8.530). Assuming a life of 20 years, the annualization factor for the treatment room is 14.877, and its annualized capital cost in the first year is US$ 360 (US$ 5000 × 1.07 = US$ 5350; US$ 5350 ÷ 14.877). Together, the annualized capital costs in the first year are US$ 1614.

The variable and fixed costs are as follows:

Variable costs:

	US$
Physician (0.25 of annual salary of US$ 10 000)	2500
Technician (0.5 of annual salary of US$ 3000)	1500
Nurse (0.5 of annual salary of US$ 5000)	2500
Supplies	4500
Total variable costs	11 000

Fixed costs:	
Annualized capital costs	1614
Maintenance	500
Administrative salaries	1000
Total fixed costs	3114
Total fixed and variable costs	14 114

3b. The new endoscopy procedure will forestall the admission of 250 surgical patients who would each have spent about a week in the hospital. Thus, the procedure will relinquish the beds that would have been occupied by these patients. As the hospital is crowded, it is likely that doctors would use the capacity in the surgical ward, operating room and recovery rooms to admit 250 "replacement" patients who, on balance, would not otherwise have been accommodated at the hospital. (The number of replacement patients assumes that they would have had the same length of stay as the former surgery patients now receiving endoscopy.) The impact on the surgical department would be twofold: saving the cost of the patients whose surgery was averted, but adding the cost of the replacement patients. If the hospital did not have a long waiting list of eligible patients, overall surgical admissions might decline.

3c. The anticipated gross revenues for the new programme would be US$ 6250 (250 diagnostic patients at US$ 25) plus US$ 12 500 (250 surgical patients at US$ 50), or US$ 18 750. The net revenues are half of this amount, or US$ 9375. Thus, the net revenues would cover about two-thirds of the costs of this programme. Several options need to be considered to cover this short-fall. First, the charge for diagnosis could be raised to US$ 38 and that for treat-ment (which forestalls a week of hospitalization) could be raised to US$ 75. Second, collections could be increased and free care reduced. Third, it might be possible to improve collections overall for the hospital. Finally, additional subsidy could be sought from the Ministry of Health.

3d. The project produces three types of health benefit. First, there is benefit to both types of endoscopy patient. Those receiving diagnosis only may obtain a more reliable diagnosis. Some patients may be spared unnecessary surgery and others will receive treatment earlier. Second, the patients receiv-ing treatment would benefit from a faster recovery and, perhaps, a lower com-plication risk. Third, replacement patients admitted to the hospital because beds are made available will enjoy an improvement in health. On balance, the new service would allow the hospital to treat 250 additional surgical patients at an annual cost of US$ 14 114, or US$ 56 per patient or US$ 8 per day. This is commensurate with or lower than the costs of many secondary hospitals in developing countries (Barnum & Kutzin, 1993). This service justifies its costs at least as much as that of other hospital services. Dr Vivek's proposal repre-sents a reasonable, though not extraordinary, programme.

3e. The annualized capital cost of US$ 1614 would not be reduced to zero from an economic viewpoint. It represents the one-year value of money invested in the capital asset of the equipment and the room renovation. The depreciation, computed by accountants, is less. Using straight-line deprecia-tion it would be US$ 1250 [US$ 10 000/(10 years) plus US$ 5000/(20 years)]. The difference between these amounts is the opportunity cost of the money invested in the project.

Answers to Exercise 4

Making decisions on which capital projects will be undertaken is not an easy task for the Ministry of Health. The ministry's challenge is to allocate limited resources to a small number of projects. Your challenge is to present the best project information possible to enable the ministry to make a deci-sion. Your part is extremely important because inadequate or inaccurate project information can lead to bad decision-making by the Ministry of Health.

Ideally, five major categories of information should be presented as part of your analysis:

Coherence with hospital and ministry goals. This is the whole rationale behind the ministry's decision-making: scarce resources are to be allocated among a virtually unlimited number of investment opportunities. The min-istry's limitation on allowable operating cost is an encouragement for you to submit only those projects that are in the hospital's best interests, and to submit those that are not in conflict with the broader goals and objectives of the ministry as a whole.

Identifying the alternatives available. Too many times, capital expenditures are presented on a "take it or leave it" basis; yet there are usually alternatives. For example, you may want to select different companies in the purchasing process to acquire the highest quality and lowest cost. Also, you may want to define different boundaries in the scope of the project over a certain time period.

Cost data. It is clear from this manual that cost information is an important variable in the capital project decision-making process. The life cycle costs of your proposed project should be presented. Limiting cost information to capital costs or operating costs can be counterproductive.

Benefit data. Benefit data can be divided into two categories: quantitative and qualitative. Quantitative information is not only synonymous with financial data but also encompasses service utilization data. Thus, it is important that your proposal includes an impact analysis that discusses the existing situation and the anticipated effects of implementing a programme.

For example, let us assume that your hospital is located in the Tansa Valley of India, a very rural area of many villages and towns. The nearest hospital that provides inpatient care in obstetrics and gynaecology is 30 miles away in Mumbai in a tertiary setting. One of the stated goals of your proposed project is to open 12 inpatient beds for obstetrical and gynaecological care, using a phased-in approach based on demonstrated demand. A realistic and quantifiable benefit of this project would be a numerical increase in patient-days for your institution and an associated increase in revenue (in some small way from paying patients). To show these benefits, you need to provide demographic data on your catchment area, including the proportion of women by certain age categories you expect to admit to your new inpatient unit. A qualitative benefit of the project is that it will allow local residents to have access to obstetrical and gynaecological care without travelling long distances.

Data regarding prior performance. Information on prior operating results of projects funded by the Ministry and/or the hospital can provide insight regarding the hospital's performance and reliability in forecasting.

Answers to Exercise 5

5a. The two pieces of information that need to be obtained from the sample are the number of invoices for unofficial drugs and the average expenditure per invoice for unofficial drugs. By multiplying these two pieces of information, one can estimate expenditures on unofficial drugs. Expenditures on official drugs had apparently already been obtained, but could be validated using the same process. These two expenditures should then be summed to obtain an estimated total amount spent on drugs during the sampling period.

5b. The first step is to choose the time period for the sample. The second step is to choose the sampling approach or method. There are several sampling approaches that can be used.

Monthly sampling: If you choose a sampling period of 12 months of a particular fiscal year, one sampling approach is to divide the invoices by month, which gives you 12 batches. From each month, randomly choose three calendar days (not necessarily regular workdays). Pull out the invoices for these three days for each month. The result is 36 batches. Some of these batches may contain no invoices if no drugs were ordered on that day. Include them anyway. Now separate the 36 batches into two piles: official and unofficial. Total each of these categories to estimate total expenditures on official drugs and total expenditures on unofficial drugs. To obtain the average amount per invoice for each category of expenditure, divide the respective total expenditure by the total number of invoices sampled for each category. To find the average number of invoices per day, divide the total count of invoices by 36. To arrive at the annual number of invoices, multiply the daily average by the number of regular workdays in the year (if the sample days were drawn only from workdays), or by the total number of calendar days in the year (365 or 366) if the days were sampled without regard to their workday status (i.e. if holidays and weekends were included).

Weekly sampling: Here the sampling units are weeks and you control for day-of-week effects. For the first week, randomly select one day by choosing a random number between 1 and 7. For each successive week, choose the next day of the week. For example, if Tuesday is selected for the first week, Wednesday would be selected for the second week, Thursday for the third, and so on. Now separate the invoices into two piles: unofficial and official. Continue the same process as for monthly sampling.

5c. This fixed-size sampling approach uses batches based on 3 centimetres rather than months or weeks. The choice of approach should be based primarily on convenience in identifying the requisite batches. In the fixed-size approach, the number of invoices per year is 2000. The value of unofficial drug purchases is estimated at US$ 210 000. This is calculated as US$ 105 per invoice multiplied by 2000 invoices. Similarly, the estimated official invoices total US$ 880 000 (calculated as US$ 440 per invoice multiplied by 2000 invoices), which means that the administrator's report of US$ 900 000 in official drug purchases is close to this approximation from the sample. Adding the official and unofficial expenditures, the total drug expenditures are US$ 1 110 000 (adding the estimated US$ 210 000 in unofficial drugs to US$ 900 000 in official drugs). The unofficial share is 18.9%.

5d. Based on a total of 12 000 hospital admissions for the most recent fiscal year, the average drug cost per admission is US$ 92.50 (US$ 1 110 000/12 000 admissions).

5e. The total cost for the three clinical services using the proportional breakdown of drug cost is as follows: US$ 366 300 (0.33 × US$ 1 110 000) for medicine wards, US$ 555 000 (0.50 × US$ 1 110 000) and US$ 188 700 (0.17 × US$ 1 110 000).

5f. Floor space is not a reliable measure of drug use. This is because drug disbursements are not a function of the area of space on a particular ward but rather of the number of patients admitted to a hospital or the number of visits to a particular clinic and the utilization by each patient. Obviously, floor space is a reliable measure for housekeeping or janitorial costs. A reasonable measure of drug use could be the number of prescriptions filled by the inpatient and outpatient pharmacy services. A sample that includes the average cost per prescription by ward would improve the estimate.

5g,h. As is shown below, the total value (price multiplied by quantity) of drugs purchased by each ward is as follows: US$ 1800 (medicine), US$ 1100 (surgery), and US$ 1050 (maternity). For this sample, each ward's share of drug costs (rounded) was 46% (medicine), 28% (surgery), and 27% (maternity).

Total value of drugs purchased by each ward (example)

Ward	Drug A (US$)	Drug B (US$)	Drug C (US$)	Total cost by ward (US$)	Ward share of total (%)
Medicine	500 (100 bottles × $5)	500 (50 bottles × $10)	800 (40 bottles × $20)	1800	45.6
Surgery	400 (80 bottles × $5)	300 (30 bottles × $10)	400 (20 bottles × $20)	1100	27.8
Maternity	350 (70 bottles × $5)	500 (50 bottles × $10)	200 (10 bottles × $20)	1050	26.6
Total cost by drug	1250	1300	1400	3950	

Using the total cost figure of US$ 1 110 000 and each ward's share of drug costs, the total drug cost by ward is the following: US$ 506 160 (0.456 × US$ 1 110 000), US$ 308 580 (0.278 × US$ 1 110 000), and US$ 295 260 (0.266 × US$ 1 110 000).

5i. Dividing each ward's drug costs by its admission volume, the drug cost per admission by ward is as follows: US$ 169 (US$ 506 160/3000), US$ 77 (US$ 308 580/4000), and US$ 59 (US$ 295 260/5000). Compared to the hospital's own drug cost estimates, which were based on official records only and allocated on the basis of each ward's share of floor space, the drug cost per medical admission is 125% more (i.e. US$ 169 rather than US$ 75). The drug cost per surgical admission is about 5% less than the hospital's estimate (US$ 77 rather than US$ 81), and the drug cost per maternity admission is about 16% less than the estimate (US$ 59 rather than US$ 70).

Comparison of pharmacy revenues using floor space allocation
versus actual purchases

Ward	Number of admissions	Method 1: total pharmacy costs using floor space allocation (US$)	Method 2: total pharmacy costs using actual purchases (US$)	Difference (method 1 minus method 2) (US$)
Medicine	3000	225 000 ($75 × 3000)	506 160 ($169 × 3000)	−281 160
Surgery	4000	324 000 ($81 × 4000)	308 580 ($77 × 4000)	15 420
Maternity	5000	351 000 ($70 × 5000)	295 260 ($59 × 5000)	55 740
Total		900 000	1 110 000	−210 000

The difference of US$ 210 000 is attributed to unofficial drugs not being accounted for by the administrator. The difference points to the inaccuracies of the hospital administrator's own estimates, both in terms of the overall average drug cost per admission and in the breakdown by each of the three wards (medical, surgical, maternity). This example also highlights the fact that the hospital administrator was erroneous in using floor space allocation as the measure of pharmacy costs.

Answers to Exercise 6

6a. Essential hospital services can be defined as those services that make a substantial contribution to the health of the people of Caribana, can be delivered at relatively low cost, and can be delivered effectively in most hospitals. Key factors in defining these services are high frequency of admission, capacity to deliver cost-effective treatments, and relatively low levels of technology (to ensure their widespread use). To operationalize these factors, it is useful to determine the leading causes of hospital admission, their cost-effectiveness (measured, in part, as the relationship between hospital costs and subsequent health improvement), and technology (measured perhaps by the proportion of the country's hospitals that can deliver the service with adequate quality).

To determine the cost of these services, some system of estimating cost by type of admission would be needed. A rough approximation would be an estimate of cost per day by type of admission (e.g. medicine, surgery, paediatrics). Then the cost of each type of admission could be estimated as the cost per day for the respective type of admission multiplied by the length of stay.

6b. A payment system must cover the hospital's reasonable and necessary costs. It should also provide incentives for economic efficiency — i.e. encourage the hospital to admit the appropriate patients and to treat them effectively and efficiently. Unfortunately, all payment systems create a mix of "positive" and "negative" incentives.

If everyone in the population selects or is assigned to a particular hospital for covered services, then each hospital could be prepaid a capitated rate (a fixed amount for each person who is enrolled or assigned with the hospital). This process ensures the hospital a flow of resources while not encouraging excessive hospitalization. Prepayment, however, creates the risk that the hospital will not provide a sufficient quantity or quality of service, either in terms of the number of persons admitted or the level of treatment provided per case.

Reimbursement on a per case basis, as used in the United States' Medicare Programme (using Diagnosis Related Groups, or DRGs), provides an incentive for cost control during the course of a hospitalization, though not on the decision about which or how many patients to admit. It also provides perverse incentives to under-provide care to keep treatment costs below reimbursement levels, and to have frequent readmissions of patients in order to receive additional case-based payments. Payment on the basis of fee-for-service induces increased quantity of treatment but is often inflationary.

Because of the mixed incentives of all payment systems, corresponding administrative systems are needed to compensate for the negative incentives. A good example is utilization review, which can be used to compare treatment (including prescribing) patterns with defined protocols, determine if admissions are justified, and so forth.

6c. Hospital costs are likely to rise from expanding reimbursement for essential services. It is likely that some areas and some persons are underserved. If non-essential drugs were previously covered, the insurance system might actually reduce the utilization of those services.

www.ingramcontent.com/pod-product-compliance
Lightning Source LLC
Chambersburg PA
CBHW081824200326

41597CB00023B/4374